Rahma Gargouri
Ben Mahmoud Lobna
Bahloul Najla

Children suspected of being allergic to beta-lactam antibiotics

Rahma Gargouri
Ben Mahmoud Lobna
Bahloul Najla

Children suspected of being allergic to beta-lactam antibiotics

Traps to avoid

ScienciaScripts

Imprint

Cover image: www.ingimage.com

This book is a translation from the original published under ISBN 978-620-6-70771-4.

Publisher:
Sciencia Scripts
is a trademark of
Dodo Books Indian Ocean Ltd. and OmniScriptum S.R.L publishing group

120 High Road, East Finchley, London, N2 9ED, United Kingdom
Str. Armeneasca 28/1, office 1, Chisinau MD-2012, Republic of Moldova, Europe
Printed at: see last page
ISBN: 978-620-8-19515-1

Thank you

A

Our teacher and jury president,

Professor JIHEN BOUGUILA

Pediatrics Department, CHU Farfat Hashed, Sousse.

A

Our teacher and jury member,

Professor SAMAH JOOBEUR

Pneumology Department, C-HU Fattouma Bourguiba, Monastir

A

Our teacher and jury member,

Associate Professor RACHIDA LAAMIRI,

Department of Pediatric Surgery, CHU Fattouma Bourguiba, Monsatir

A

My memory directors:

Mrs Lo6na Ben Mahmoud

University Professor

Sfaχ Regional Pharmacology Department

Mrs Salma Ben Ameur

University Professor

Department of Pediatrics CHU Hédi Cheker Sfaχ

We thank you for agreeing to supervise and evaluate this work, and for your interest in it. You have our deepest gratitude.

Table of contents

INTRODUCTION

Allergic disease is one of the most common chronic pathologies according to the WHO, and is on the increase. Allergic reactions account for a third of all adverse drug reactions (1). The drugs most often blamed are antibiotics, particularly beta-lactam antibiotics. Numerous studies have shown that only 15% of patients said to be allergic to a drug are actually allergic (2,3). In fact, there is often a contrast between people who are really allergic and those who believe they are, due to the occurrence of symptoms mistaken for hypersensitivity. The most typical example is infectious mononucleosis, which is often accompanied by a skin rash after taking amoxicillin, without there being any allergy (4). What's alarming is that this over-diagnosis of allergy is causing a therapeutic restriction for certain reference treatments in many common pathologies, notably ENT and pulmonary. What's more, the use of alternative molecules, often with a broader spectrum, disturbs the microbiota, creating resistance. The medical side of the problem is accompanied by a financial one. Indeed, several studies have highlighted the increased cost of infection in so-called allergic subjects (5,6).

One example is the beta-lactam family, which includes penicillins, cephalosporins, carbapenems and other lesser-used molecules. This family poses the problem not only of allergy, but also of cross-allergy. Indeed, these molecules are synthesized from a common core to prevent resistance, but present differences within their side chains. It is therefore important to distinguish between an allergy to the beta-lactam cycle, which implies a ban on all molecules in this family, and an allergy to a side chain, in which case a single molecule is banned. The notion of cross-allergies between penicillins and cephalosporins should therefore be taken into consideration (7).

These problems of allergy, cross-allergy and false allergy, with all the prescribing limitations they engender, pose a greater problem in the infection-prone paediatric population.

In fact, β-lactams broaden the antibacterial spectrum, with good tissue diffusion, the possibility of administration via the digestive tract for some molecules, and even the possibility of dose spacing. This makes β-lactams a real therapeutic advance in childhood infections (8). For example, amoxicillin is the antibiotic of choice against pneumococcus, group A streptococcus and Haemophilus influenzae. This spectrum makes it one of the best weapons in pediatrics in over two-thirds of cases. The prescription of macrolides as an alternative runs up against the risk of resistance, and the prescription of second- or third-generation oral cephalosporins is hampered by their poorer microbiological activity (9).

This is the background to our work, the aim of which was to study the characteristics of a paediatric population referred to the Sfax regional pharmacovigilance service for suspected betalactam allergy.

PATIENTS AND METHODS

I. TYPE OF STUDY

This is a cross-sectional, monocentric, descriptive study based on a population of children consulting the regional pharmacovigilance service, which is located at the Sfax Faculty of Medicine, for suspected allergy to betalactam antibiotics. These children were referred to the service by another physician. The study was spread over two years, from January 2020 to December 2022.

II. STUDY POPULATION

- Patient inclusion criteria were as follows:
  - Children up to the age of 15, referred to the regional pharmacovigilance service for suspected adverse reactions, with at least one drug belonging to the betalactam class.
  - Patients included in this study have a descriptive report of the event, and a pharmacovigilance file containing sufficient information for the study to be carried out.
- The exclusion criteria are:
  - Children referred for suspected non-drug allergies.
  - Children referred for suspected allergy to drugs other than beta-lactam antibiotics.
  - Incomplete files.

III. DATA COLLECTION

The data required for this study were collected from the pharmacovigilance archive. A data collection form was specially designed for this work. (appendix 1) The data collected are :

- Socio-demographic data: age, gender
- Pathological history and terrain :
  - Non-allergic pathological history and acute and chronic medications taken
  - Allergic history: personal and family atopy (atopic dermatitis, rhinoconjunctivitis, asthma), and history of drug intolerance.
- Data concerning the adverse event
  - The nature of the antibiotic, presumed to be allergenic, belonging to the beta-lactam family, at the time of the current event, the INN, and the reason for its prescription (ENT causes, abscess, etc.).
  - The nature of the event: cutaneous and extra-cutaneous lesions, signs of severity. Cutaneous involvement was described according to its topography, nature and pruritic character.
  - For cases of typical acute urticaria, severity was established according to the Ring and Ressmer classification (10) (appendix 2).
  - Chronology of the event:
    - ✓ The time between the suspected allergic reaction and the consultation, the time between taking the medication and the clinical manifestations, and the day the medication was taken.
    - ✓ Symptoms on discontinuation and/or continuation of treatment
- Imputability score calculation: The imputability score is calculated at the Sfax Regional Pharmacovigilance Department using the French Bégaud method. This method is based on the calculation of the intrinsic imputability score from chronology (time of onset, evolution after

cessation of treatment) and semiology, and is also based on a bibliographic score. At the end of this calculation, a global imputability score was also evaluated. Details of how these scores were calculated are summarized in Appendix 3. (11) (appendix 3).

- Results of allergological investigation if performed: In patients who received an allergological investigation, the data from the latter were collected from their records:
  - Skin tests were carried out with the informed consent of patients' relatives, eliminating contraindications, complying with patient safety rules and in accordance with the recommendations of the European Network on Drug Allergy/European Academy of Allergy and Clinical Immunology (ENDA/EAACI): (12)
    - ✓ The time of onset was considered the first means of differentiating the mechanisms of hypersensitivity: if the reaction occurred within an hour of exposure, the immediate origin was evoked. If the reaction occurred more than one hour after exposure, a delayed origin was more likely(12).
    - ✓ In the event of a suspected Ig E-mediated immediate hypersensitivity reaction (anaphylaxis, urticaria, angioedema, bronchospasm, runny nose, red eyes, etc.), skin tests (prick test ± immediate-read IDR) were performed as a first-line treatment.
    - ✓ If a delayed reaction was suspected (maculo- papular exanthema, fixed erythema, photoallergic reaction, ...), patch tests (± delayed-reading RID) were then performed.

Readings were taken at 72 hours, and not until three hours after the patch had been opened, to eliminate maceration-related artifacts as far as possible. (13)

Interpretation of the tests and comparison with the clinical history made it possible to classify the patient in one of two situations:

- Positive skin tests confirm allergy: molecule banned.
- Negative skin tests with suggestion of an oral provocation test (OPT).

A patient was considered allergic to one or more betalactam antibiotics if the skin tests were positive or if the oral provocation test was positive. (14)

IV. STATISTICAL DATA

This is a cross-sectional, descriptive study.

Data entry and statistical analysis were carried out using the 20th version of SPSS (Statistical Package for the Social Sciences) software.

We recorded all the characteristics of the study population. Quantitative variables were described using means and extreme values. Qualitative variables were described using proportions and translated into figures or tables.

RESULTS

This study included 38 children presenting with suspected beta-lactam allergy. Data relating to patients, drug intake, adverse reaction and allergological investigation were detailed:

I. PATIENT DEMOGRAPHICS AND ANTECEDENTS

1. Age

The mean age of our population was 5.5 ±3.8 years, with extremes ranging from 3 months to 13 years.

2. Type

Males predominated (N= 23, 60.5%), with an M/F sex ratio of 1.53.

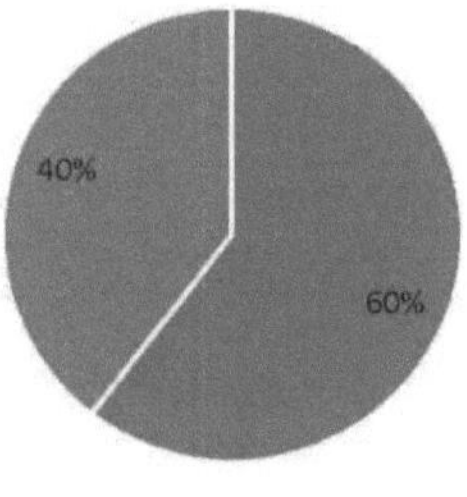

Figure 1: Distribution of children by gender

3. Pathological history of patients

3.1. Allergological history

In our population, there was no family or personal history of drug allergy. Only one case of dermographism was noted. No documented history of chronic urticaria or food allergy was noted. Atopy was noted in 5 children (13.15%). Asthma was noted in two children (5.26%).

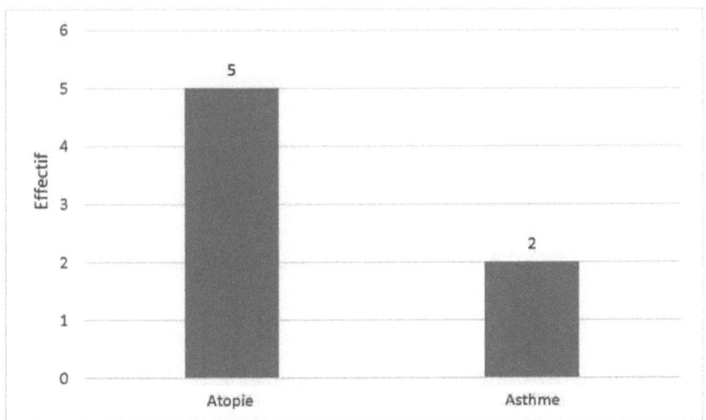

Figure 2: Distribution of allergological histories in the study population

3.2 Non-allergic history

In our population, a trisomy 21 atrial septal defect was noted in one child for whom no medication was received. Acute lymphocytic leukemia was also reported in a child not yet on anticancer treatment.

II. CHARACTERISTICS OF THE PRESUMED ALLERGIC REACTION

1 Nature of the reaction

Cutaneous signs were the most frequent manifestation in N=32 children (84.2%), followed by respiratory signs in N=4 children (10.5%).

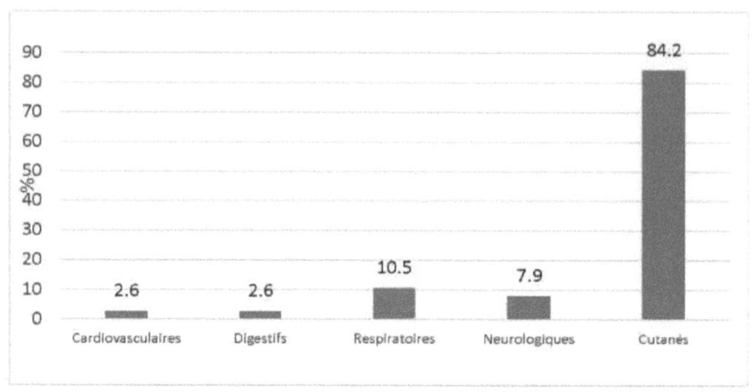

Figure 3: Symptoms presented by patients during an adverse event

1.1. Skin reactions

Skin lesions were pruritic in N=24 cases (63.15%). Typical urticaria was diagnosed in 20 children (52.6%). Typical maculopapular exanthema was noted in 7 patients (18.4%). The skin involvement concerned the whole body in N=28 cases (73.63%). Only one case of angioedema was associated with urticaria.

Table 1: Skin lesions present in the study population at the time of the suspected allergic adverse event

	Workforce	Percentage
Pruritus		
Pruritic lesion	**24**	**63,15**
Non-pruritic lesion	**8**	**21,05**
Lesion site		
Trunk lesions	**2**	**5,26**
Limb lesions	**2**	**5,26**
Generalized lesions	**28**	**73,63**
Type of lesion		
Urticaria	**20**	**52,6**
Maculopapular exanthema	**7**	**18,4**
Non-specific skin rush	**5**	**13**
Angioedema	**1**	**2,6**

1.2. Extracutaneous reactions

Cardiovascular signs

Mottling with cyanosis was noted in only one patient (2.6%).

Respiratory signs

Respiratory discomfort was reported by 4 patients (10.5%). Wheezing was noted in only one case (2.6%).

Neurological signs

Neurological signs were present in 3 patients (7.9%):

A chewing reaction and hypertonia were observed in a patient on cefotaxime, accompanied by cyanosis. These were the only signs of stage 3 anaphylaxis in this patient.

Two cases of loss of consciousness were also reported.

Digestive signs

Digestive signs were noted in just one patient (2.6%), with abdominal pain mistaken for anaphylaxis, and elevated pancreatic enzymes in a child taking ceftazidime.

1.3. Immediate hypersensitivity

Immediate hypersensitivity was reported in N=21 patients (55.26% of the study population). According to the Ring and Messmer classification, the majority of cases were stage 1, with typical urticarial lesions. One case of angioedema was noted in a child.

A stage 2 was noted in one patient with urticaria and wheezing dyspnea.

Stage 3 anaphylaxis with cyanosis, mottling, chewing and hypertonia of the limbs was observed in a patient without typical urticaria.

Table 2: Distribution of HSI cases according to the Ring and Messmer staging system

Stage of anaphylaxis	Urticaria lesion N (%)	No urticarial lesions N (%)	Total N (%)
Stage 1	19 (50)	0	19 (50)
Stage 2	1 (2,6)	0	1 (2,6)
Stage 3	0	1(2,6)	1 (2,6)
Stage 4	0	0	0

1.4. Delayed hypersensitivity

Of the 13 cases in which the time to onset of symptoms was accurately recorded, 9 patients (69%) had a delayed onset of symptoms beyond one hour.

In the study population, typical maculopapular exanthema was identified in 7 patients, i.e. 18.4% of cases.

2 Severity of reaction

Among cases of immediate hypersensitivity, severe reactions were noted in 3 children, including one case of angioedema, one case of stage 2 anaphylaxis (respiratory signs) and another of stage 3 (neurological and cardiovascular signs).

Among the cases of delayed hypersensitivity, there were no cases of severe lesions.

3.location of reaction

In more than half the cases (61%), the adverse reaction occurred at home.

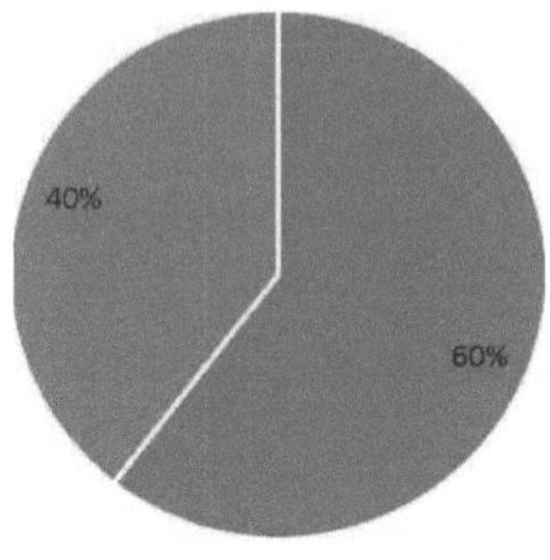

Figure 4: Location of suspected allergic reaction in the study population

III. DIETARY AND DRUG EXPOSURE AT THE UNDESIRABLE EVENT

l.Medicines

At the time of the adverse event, medication other than beta-lactam antibiotics was documented in more than half the cases (N=20, 52.6%).

1.1 Antibiotics

1.1.1 Betalactam prescription regimen

1.1.1.1 The molecule

Amoxicillin was the molecule most frequently received by patients in the study population (39.5%). 3rd-generation cephalosporins were received in 34.2% of cases.

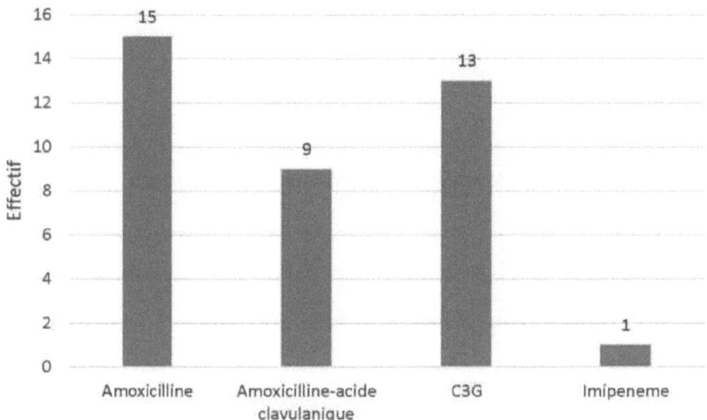

Figure 5: List of betalactam antibiotics received by patients during the presumed allergic reaction

The 3rd generation cephalosporins most frequently reported were cefotaxime (157%), and ceftriaxone (10.52%). Two cases received oral cefixime, including one conversion to the injectable form.

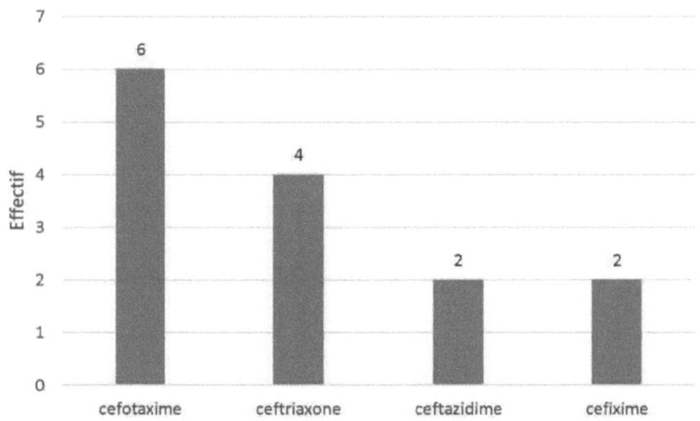

Figure 6: 3rd generation cephalosporins received by the study population during the presumed allergic reaction

1.1.1.2 Previous betalactam sensitization

On questioning the patients and especially their relatives, the notion of previous sensitization to the accused drug was confirmed in 5 cases

(13.15%), and denied in 8 others (21%). Information was lacking in 65.7% of cases.

1.1.1.3 Betalactam administration route

In N=25 cases (66%), the children had received the antibiotic orally. The intravenous route was reported in 26% of cases.

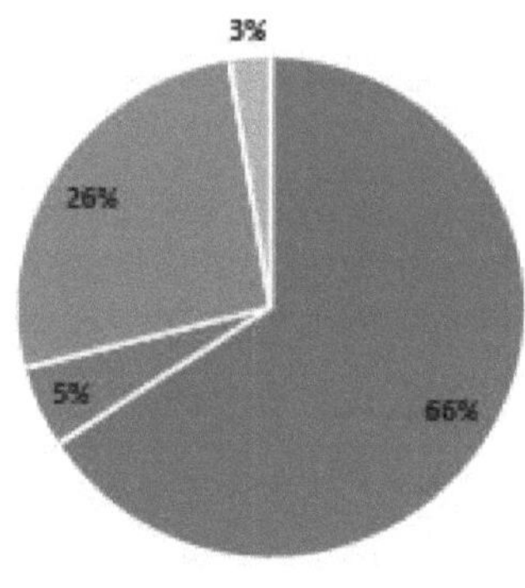

Figure 7: Routes of beta-lactam administration in the study population

1.1.1.4 Reason for prescribing beta-lactam antibiotics

In 20 cases (54%), the reason for prescribing betalactam was not explicitly mentioned in the patients' files. An ENT cause was most frequently reported in N=11 cases (28.9%). A urinary tract infection was noted in one patient, and renal abscesses were observed in another.

All pathologies combined, concomitant fever was noted in N=24 patients (62.3%). Influenza-like illness was reported in only 3 cases (7.9%).

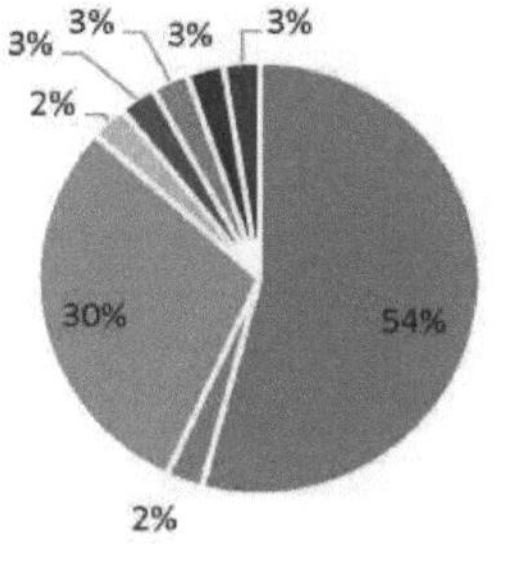

Figure 8: Reasons for prescribing betalactam antibiotics in the study population

1.1.2 Non-betalactam antibiotics

Antibiotic therapy was prescribed concomitantly with beta-lactam antibiotics in N=9 patients (23.7%).

The molecule most frequently used was vancomycin in 4 patients (10.52%). Piperacillin-tazobactam" was recommended for one patient, combined with metronidazole. Gentamycin and rovamycin were co-prescribed in just one patient each.

1.2. Non-antibiotic drugs

At the time of the suspected allergic reaction, paracetamol was the most co-prescribed molecule in N=8 (21.1%), followed by NSAIDs and corticoids in N=4 (10.5%) each. No consumption of

neuroleptics or tricyclic antidepressants.

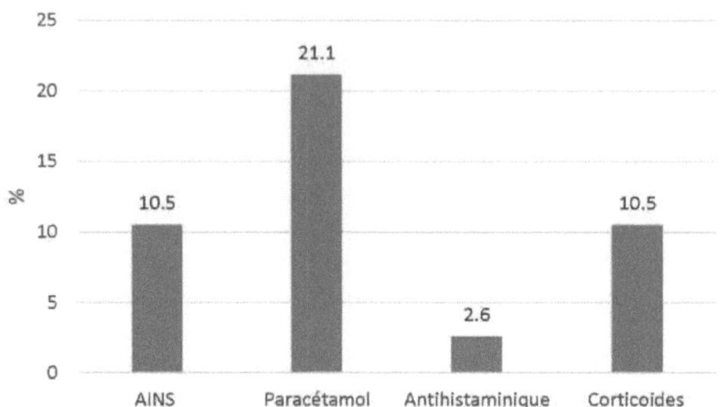

Figure 9: Distribution of medications taken at the time of the adverse event

2. Food intake

Consumption of a chocolate-type histaminolytic agent on the day of the event was reported in only one patient.

Seafood consumption was reported in two children.

IV. IMPUTABILITY

1.Chronological imputability

1.1 Delay

1.1.1 Time between adverse reaction and pharmacovigilance consultation

The average time elapsed between the incident and the pharmacovigilance consultation was 118 days ±179, with extremes ranging from 2 to 700 days.

1.1.2 Time between start of betalactam treatment and occurrence of adverse reaction

The mean duration of betalactam treatment up to the occurrence of the adverse event was 4.5 days ±6.1, with extremes ranging from 1 to 20 days. However, this detail was only specified in 20 files.

1.1.3 Time between last medication and occurrence of adverse reaction

The average time elapsed between the last medication taken and the adverse reaction was 3.7 hours ±4.03, with extremes ranging from 6 minutes to 12 hours. However, this detail was only accurately specified in 13 files.

This delay was less than or equal to one hour, indicating an immediate reaction in 4 (31%) patients, and greater than one hour, indicating a delayed reaction in 9 (69%).

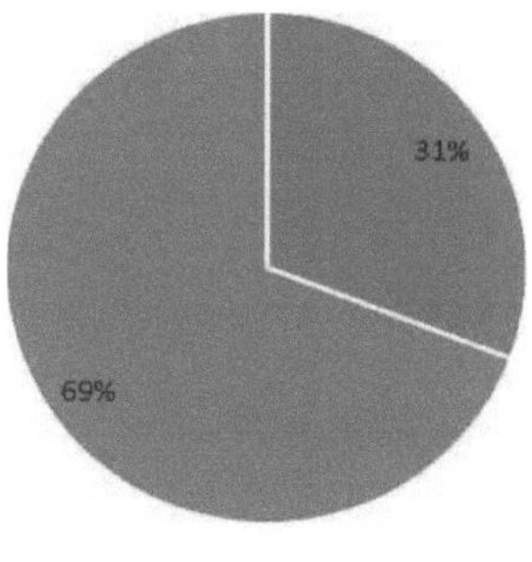

Figure 10: Time to onset of adverse reaction in relation to drug intake

1.2. Evolution of clinical manifestations of the adverse event

After symptomatic treatment and discontinuation of antibiotic therapy, the clinical manifestations resolved in 34 patients (89.47%). A recurrence of the maculopapular rash was noted even after discontinuation of treatment in one atopic child. On the other hand, in 4 other patients, continuity of treatment had no influence on the symptoms, which also developed favorably.

1.3. Chronological score

According to the French Bégaud method, chronological imputability was doubtful in N=18 patients (47%), and plausible in N=17 others (45%). It was probable in only two patients.

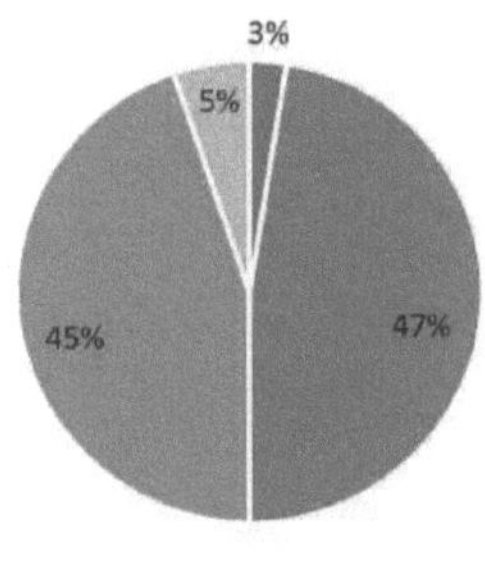

Figure 11: Interpretation of chronological imputability scores in the study population

2. semiological imputability

According to the French Bégaud method, semiological imputability was doubtful in half the cases (N=19). It was probable in only one patient.

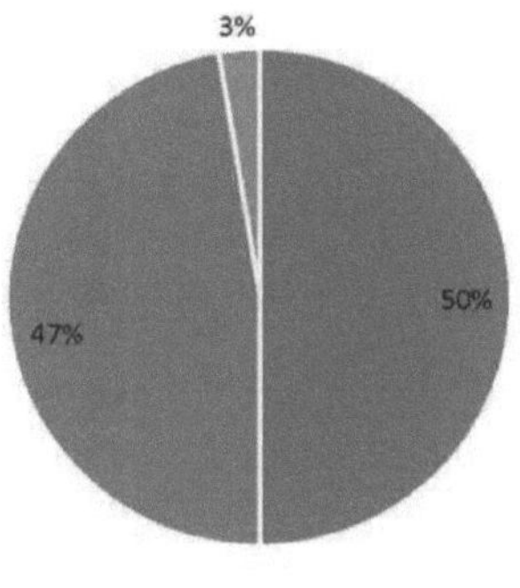

Figure 12: Interpretation of semiological imputability scores in the study population

Differential diagnoses were evoked in the case of skin lesions with doubtful semiological imputability (S1). These included infection N= 21 (55%), allergy to other concomitant treatments N=4 (10.5%), food allergy following seafood consumption N=2 (5.26%), and histaminoliberation in an atopic patient who had consumed chocolate (2.6%).

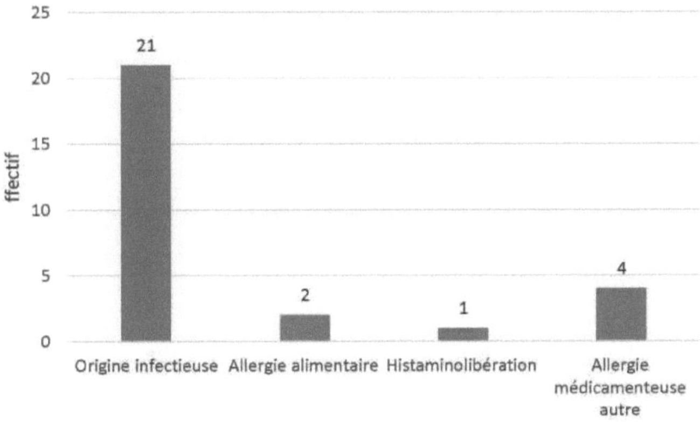

Figure 13: Differential diagnoses advanced by the pharmacovigilance survey for skin lesions in the study population with a semiological score of S1

Among patients who finally underwent allergological investigation, a semiological imputability level (S3) with positive results was rectified in N=3 patients (7.89%). Apart from cutaneous manifestations, one case of abdominal pain was mistaken for anaphylaxis, and ultimately attributed to pancreatic damage. A case of purely biological hepatic disturbance was reported with a suspected DRESS syndrome, and cytolysis at 31 times normal was noted in a patient on ceftazidime.

3. Calculation of the Intrinsic imputability score

Intrinsic imputability was doubtful in N=25 cases (65.78%). It was probable in only one patient.

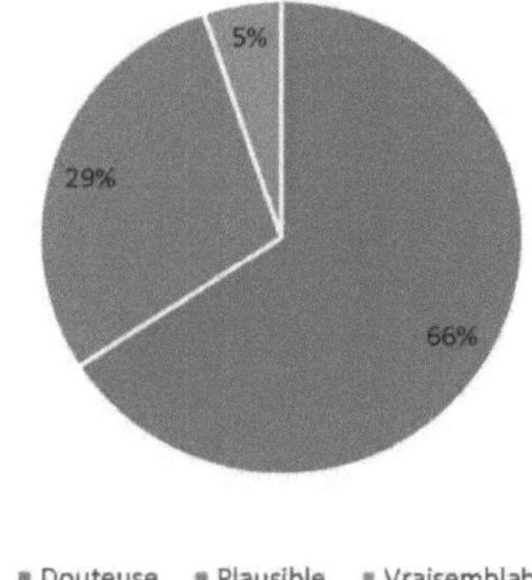

Figure 14: Interpretation of intrinsic imputability scores in the study population

4.bibliographical imputability

In terms of the literature, beta-lactams had a notable effect in relation to the reactions described by all our patients.

5 Overall interpretation of the imputability score

In 63.15% of cases (N=24), the overall imputability of the adverse reaction to the drug was doubtful. It was probable in 3 patients (8%).

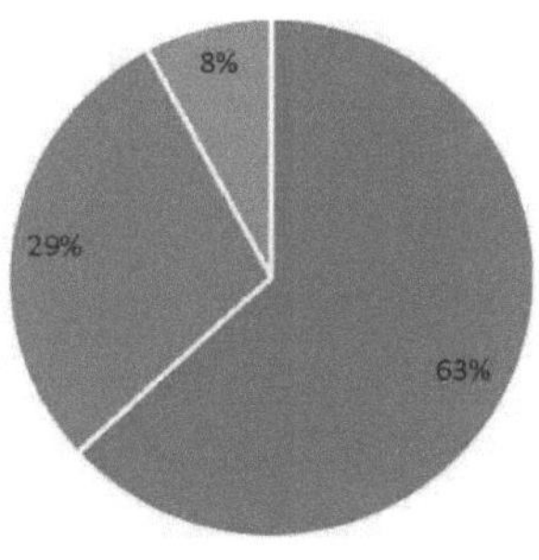

Figure 15: Overall interpretation of imputability scores for the study population

Allergological investigation was indicated in 14 patients (36.84% of cases). Supervised drug intake was authorized in 14 other patients. Discontinuation of the indication for investigation was noted in 10 patients, including two cases where the imputability of the reaction to drug intake was probable, and 4 cases where it was plausible (Table 3).

In the 3 cases where imputability was probable, reintroduction of the drug was prohibited from the outset (Table 3).

In cases where imputability was plausible, use of the same drug involved in the reaction was prohibited. If necessary, two cases were authorized to take another betalactamine under supervision, 4 cases were not, and 5 cases were recommended for further allergological investigation (Table 3).

In cases where imputability was doubtful, betalactam use was authorized under supervision in 31.57% of cases. Unrestricted and unconditional authorization was granted in 10.52% of cases. In 21% of cases, the use of beta-lactams was forbidden, with allergological investigation proposed (Table 3).

Table 3: Distribution of study population according to imputability score and pharmacovigilance decision

Decision / Imputability score	Need for allergological investigation N (%)	No survey N (%)	Betalactam use under supervision N (%)	Total N (%)
Doubtful	8 (21)*	4 (10,52)*	12 (31,57)*	24 (63,15)
Plausible	5 (13,15)**	4 (10,52)**	2 (5,26) **	11 (28,94)
Likely	1 (2,6)	2 (5,26)	0 (0)	3 (7,86)
Total	14 (36,84)	10 (26,31)	14 (36,84)	38 (100)

* Resumption of all beta-lactam antibiotics

** Authorized use of a betalactamine other than the one taken at the time of the adverse reaction

V. ALLERGOLOGICAL SURVEY

Allergological investigations were carried out in only 6 children, i.e. 15.78% of cases.

- **For delayed reactions:**

Patch tests were used to diagnose allergy to amoxicillin + clavulanic acid in a patient who had tested positive for this compound and negative for cefpodoxime and cefuroxime. C2G and C3G were authorized. It should be noted that the overall imputability score for this case was likely.

In addition, the amoxicillin patch test was negative in two other children whose drug liability was doubtful.

- **For immediate reactions:**

A prick test was performed on 3 children:

- A patient who developed urticaria while taking amoxicillin (with doubtful overall imputability): The prick test was negative.

  - ❖ A TPO complement was performed and was negative, thus

eliminating the allergy.

- A girl who developed urticaria while receiving cefotaxime (with plausible overall imputability): The prick test was negative for amoxicillin clavulanic acid and C1G. It was doubtful for other cephalosporins. An immediate-reading TST was performed for cephalosporins and was positive for C3G.
- An asthmatic and atopic boy who developed urticaria while receiving amoxicillin clavulanic acid and C3G (with probable overall imputability): the prick test was clearly positive for amoxicillin clavulanic acid and C1G, and doubtful for C3G. But given the occurrence of an asthma attack, a cephalosporin TST was not performed, and the test was considered positive where all beta-lactam antibiotics were banned.

Table 4: Details and results of allergological survey

Patients with allergological investigations Sex(age)	Type of reaction	Betalactamine consumed	Survey results
Boy (age 7)	EMP	amoxicillin + clavulanic acid	Positive patch test for amoxicillin + clavulanic acid Patch test negative for cefpodoxime and cefuroxime
Boy (1 year)	EMP	amoxicillin	Negative patch test
Girl (5 years)	EMP	amoxicillin	Negative patch test
Boy (age 7)	Urticaria	amoxicillin + clavulanic acid and C3G (cefotaxime)	Prick test positive for amoxicillin clavulanic acid and C1G and doubtful for C3G + asthma attack
Girl (8 years)	Urticaria	C3G (cefotaxime)	Prick test negative for amoxicillin clavulanic acid and C1G. Prick test doubtful for other cephalosporins. Immediate-reading TST positive for C3G.
Girl	Urticaria	Amoxicillin	Prick test negative Negative TPO

DISCUSSION

I. CLINICAL FORMS ACCORDING TO PATHOPHYSIOLOGICAL MECHANISM

l.Immediate hypersensitivity

1.1. Urticaria and angioedema

Like all urticaria, drug-induced urticaria is compensated by erythematous, edematous, patchy, geographically-contoured, migratory and fleeting papules, with pruritus.

The angioedema that sometimes accompanies it is an edema of the hypodermis and dermis under tension. Skin color is unchanged, with no pruritus. This phenomenon can affect both the skin and the mucous membranes. Seriousness lies in the involvement of the oropharynx, with the risk of asphyxia. (17)

In our series, only one case of angioedema was described without respiratory difficulty.

1.2 Anaphylaxis and anaphylactic shock

This is a serious, life-threatening accident. It follows the release of histamine from basophils and mast cells, and leukotrienes (15,16). Mucocutaneous signs are the first to appear, followed by hemodynamic distress and even cardiocirculatory arrest. Respiratory discomfort may also occur, leading to life-threatening bronchospasm.

The Ring and Rassmer classification distinguishes 4 grades of severity (10) (appendix 2). It is essentially used for immediate therapeutic decisions, but also for deciding whether to carry out an allergological investigation. This is a therapeutic emergency. The offending drug must be banned. Rapid filling must be performed, accompanied by intramuscular or intravenous administration of adrenaline. The prognosis is sometimes unfortunate. In our series, a case of cyanosis with signs of hypoperfusion was observed in a child, warranting treatment by the EMS team.

2. Delayed hypersensitivity: Toxidermia

Unlike immediate hypersensitivity, delayed drug hypersensitivity presents a wide variety of clinical pictures. It is important to know how to distinguish between the different types of toxidermia, as mortality varies according to the clinical picture, and the danger of drug rechallenge can, in some forms, be life-threatening (17).

2.1. Maculopapular exanthema (MPE)

This is the most common form of toxidermia. It is characterized by pinkish-red macules and papules, with the possibility of a slightly urticarial or purpuric appearance. The main differential diagnosis is infectious, but the polymorphism of the lesions, the pruritus, the absence of enanthema, and the absence of fever support the diagnosis. Hepatic involvement is also possible. In addition to viruses, toxin-induced exanthems can be confusing, especially in children. These tend to be scarlatiniform, accentuating on the folds and confluent, with no intervals of normal skin (17). To the touch, lesions are rough with secondary desquamation. In our series, maculopapular exanthema was diagnosed in 7 patients, while other non-specific eruptions were observed in 5 children (13%). In these cases, the infectious origin was rightly evoked in view of the distribution to the limbs, the fever and the flu-like syndrome.

The fever argument isn't very strong, since even allergic reactions can be accompanied by fever, but in most cases it's moderate. In addition, fever is common in children with bacterial infections for whom antibiotic therapy has been indicated.

Thus, the existence of a high fever alone does not rule out the likelihood of allergy. (17)

The appearance of the rash is sometimes tremulous, and may even be urticarial in the case of EMP, leading to confusion with HSI. However, the delay in onset and the possibility of other respiratory, digestive and ENT signs may help to correct the diagnosis. In the same way, true urticaria may not have a typical appearance, and may be so discreet as to be noticed at a late stage, particularly in patients already taking antihistamines or oral corticosteroids for other reasons. This situation can be quite common in atopic children. In our series, antihistamines were taken in 2.6% of cases, and systemic corticosteroids were prescribed prior to the adverse event in 10.5% of cases, which could attenuate the allergic symptomatology, particularly type I symptoms. These situations are common in the paediatric population.

2.2. Fixed erythema pigmentosum

In all cases, toxidermia is the result of taking a drug. It occurs less than 48 hours after taking the drug. Symptoms include pruritus or burning, with the appearance of erythematous, purplish, edematous papules with the possibility of bullae. The site is mainly periorificial. When the drug is reintroduced, old lesions may be reactivated, which is a major diagnostic factor. (17) No cases of erythema pigmentosum were reported in our series.

2.3 Acute generalized exanthematous pustulosis (AGEP)

It manifests as small, non-follicular pustules, with erythema, mostly on the trunk and major folds. Edema of the face and hands is also possible, as is edema of the mouth. The fever is high in this form, with a biological inflammatory syndrome that can be confused with a bacterial origin. This form manifests rapidly after treatment, and resolves spontaneously in less than 15 days, leaving a scaly appearance.(17) In this series, no cases were identified.

2.4 Stevens-Johnson and Lyell syndromes

These are pathologies in which the patient presents a skin detachment with bullae, after pressure on apparently healthy skin. Nonspecific signs may precede the cutaneous symptoms by a few days, such as fever, angina, etc. The onset of symptoms may take a few weeks longer than the time of consumption.

Stevens-Johnson syndrome manifests as erythematous lesions, sometimes associated with purpura. Mucous membranes may also be affected. Detachments do not exceed 10% of body surface area.

Lyell syndrome involves bullae and epidermal detachment, with a higher percentage of cutaneous detachment. Skin lesions spread rapidly, resembling wet linen. Mucosal lesions in the form of ulceration and necrosis are well documented. Visceral involvement is possible. The risk of death is high. This is a very serious form of the disease, the management of which would be the prerogative of specialists. (17)These severe HSR reactions were not present in our patients.

2.5 DRESS (Drug Reaction with Eosinophilia and Systemic Symptoms).

This reaction occurs a few weeks after the start of treatment. There is a pruritic maculopapular rash. Edema of the face and neck may also occur.

Certain mucous membranes may be affected, and secondary lymphoid organs may become enlarged. Fever is often responsible for a deterioration in the patient's general condition. Other visceral disorders are also possible. Recovery is slow. In our series, DRESS was suspected in the presence of acute hepatitis, but remained unlikely in the absence of hypereosinophilia.

2.6 Exceptional toxicidermia

- Photo-allergic reactions: erythematous, prominent lesions, sometimes eczematiform, extending to areas accessible to sunlight, occurring between one and 3 weeks after taking the drug. Delays are shorter in cases of re-exposure.
- Drug-induced vascular purpura: Purpuric lesions are
  painful, with the possibility of detachment. They are mainly located in the lower limbs. (17)

II. DIAGNOSTIC MANAGEMENT OF BETALACTAM HYPERSENSITIVITY

Ideally, drug allergy tests should be carried out between the 3rd month and the 2nd year following the reaction. In any case, a minimum delay of 6 weeks should be respected (17,18), especially in the case of immediate reactions, as there is a risk of false negatives. Immediate and non-immediate hypersensitivity are investigated differently, since their immunological mechanisms are not the same. To this end, the " European Network for Drug Allergy" or ENDA has produced decision trees to aid diagnostic decision-making (17,19) (appendix 4).

1. Importance of the history in the diagnosis of drug hypersensitivity

The history should be the first step in investigating drug hypersensitivity. It is one of the most sensitive and specific elements, almost as important as skin tests. It enables us to define the imputability of the drug. It is advisable to use intrinsic and extrinsic criteria identified through questioning. (17,20, 21)

Intrinsic imputability concerns the patient's history, in an attempt to establish a causal relationship between a drug and the occurrence of an adverse event. It takes into account chronological criteria such as the time between taking the drug and the occurrence of the incident, the evolution of symptoms after discontinuation of treatment, and any accidental intake of the allergen. It also considers semiological criteria. (22,23, 24)

Extrinsic imputability deals with the consistency of the allergic hypothesis with the literature.

Detailed questioning is necessary to characterize the type of initial reaction and guide the investigations to be ordered. The EDNA has validated a questionnaire covering the main data required in the event of a hypersensitivity accident (17) (appendix 5).

In our series, in cases of doubtful imputability, a decision was taken on the possibility of taking all betalactam antibiotics without further allergological investigation in 16 patients, 12 of whom were authorized to take all betalactam antibiotics with simple monitoring when taking the drug involved in the current episode, and 4 authorized to take them without restriction. This finding underlines the importance of questioning, which enables the restriction on prescribing to be lifted, allowing free therapeutic choice without the need for allergological testing.

In the event of plausible imputability, the drug involved in the adverse event is banned. On the basis of history alone, 6 patients were exempted from undergoing allergological investigation, 2 of whom were authorized to take betalactamines other than the drug involved in the current reaction under supervision, and 4 of whom were authorized to consume them without special supervision.

In cases of probable imputability, 2 patients were banned from receiving beta-lactam antibiotics, without even having to resort to an investigation. The rationale for such a decision is largely based on clinical evidence and consideration of the risk of cross-allergy.

Given the same level of imputability, the pharmacologist's decision as to whether or not to carry out an allergological investigation will depend on the molecule taken at the time of the current event, previous history of drug allergy, the existence of dermographism, the need for long-term corticosteroid treatment for another reason, and finally the logistical availability to carry out the tests. The time factor is also decisive, since allergological tests must be carried out within a minimum period of 6 weeks of the incident (17).

It should be pointed out that the importance of questioning does not lie solely in the interview with the pharmacologist or allergist.

Indeed, involving pharmacists in cases of suspected beta-lactam allergy could be part of the solution to the problem of over-diagnosis . With this in mind, a study was carried out on pharmacist involvement in patients with a notion of delayed allergy to penicillins, in which 250 patients were included. On the basis of pharmacist questioning alone, 160 suspicions were rejected. (25)

1.1 Importance of time to onset and disappearance of symptoms in defining the type of hypersensitivity

Among the valuable and decisive elements revealed by questioning is the time of onset and disappearance of the reaction in relation to the last drug taken: the picture of an immediate allergy often includes manifestations appearing within an hour of exposure, but this depends on the route of administration (oral, intravenous). Some authors have argued that it would be more logical to reconsider this delay and extend it to two hours after exposure. HSI classically involves acute urticaria and pruritus, resolving within 24 hours(12, 17).

If clinical signs persist for more than 24 hours, the diagnosis of HSI must be questioned, although atypical cases do exist. In our study, cases of urticaria were typical in terms of onset and resolution.

The picture of delayed hypersensitivity is less obvious because of the clinical diversity of toxidermia and the multitude of other possible pictures. Differential diagnoses, notably infectious ones, are very frequently found in the paediatric population. In all cases, however, symptoms appear more than an hour after exposure.

1.2 Importance of semiological analysis of symptoms to deduce pathophysiological mechanism and decide on further exploration

1.2.1 Immediate hypersensitivity

The typical urticarial nature of lesions in an allergic context is highly suggestive of immediate hypersensitivity. The severity that may accompany it is defined by hospitalization, intervention by the EMS team, or the need for adrenaline. This severity requires an allergological evaluation (17).

The same diagnostic value is attributed to the notion of an asthmatic attack or loss of consciousness, which could sometimes be the only indicators of an anaphylactic reaction. In our series, stage 3 anaphylaxis was not accompanied by urticarial lesions in one child. Another case of loss of consciousness was noted in a patient, but anaphylaxis was not considered. Imputability was deemed highly doubtful, and the drug was authorized for use if necessary, subject to monitoring.

This being said, it should be remembered that in the case of mild reactions, non-pruritic skin lesions exclude urticaria by definition. (17). Moreover, in our series, we counted 5 cases of non-specific cutaneous rush due to the absence of pruritus, and the absence of belonging to a particular semiological entity. In these cases, viral and/or atopic origin seemed the most plausible cause.

1.2.2. Delayed hypersensitivity

Sometimes the allergic mechanism of a delayed reaction is not obvious (e.g. hepatitis, vasculitis, ...), but the life-threatening nature of the reaction justifies an allergological work-up. In our series, none of the delayed reactions were serious.

Maculopapular exanthema is one of the most common toxidermia associated with HSR accidents. (26)

Frequent benign toxidermia, such as maculopapular exanthema, is contrasted with severe toxidermia, such as bullous toxidermia (17,27).

In our series, 7 cases of maculopapular exanthema were found. Patch tests were performed for 3 of them. Only one test was positive for amoxicillin clavulanic acid and negative for cephalosporins.

A suspected DRESS syndrome was noted in a patient with cytolysis greater than 30 times the norm. But patch tests were not performed. Ceftazidime was contraindicated, since it was the cause. Other cephalosporins were authorized under supervision.

2. Place of additional allergological tests

The predictive value of questioning, which remains a cornerstone of the diagnostic process, varies from 17% to 46% (28), depending on the study, demonstrating the importance of allergological investigations in specialized settings.

2.1 Skin tests

The choice of allergological tests depends on the patient's history and clinical manifestations. If immediate hypersensitivity is suspected, immediate-reading tests such as prick tests and the intradermal reaction (IDR) are indicated. On the other hand, if delayed hypersensitivity is suspected, delayed-reading tests such as patch tests and/or delayed-reading IDR are indicated. Once the skin tests have been completed, the decision is made whether or not to add an Oral Provocation Test (OPT). Initially, skin tests are performed with amoxicillin (Appendix 3) (Figure 17).

According to the literature, the practice of allergological testing for beta-lactam antibiotics is not really standardized, with variability in the molecules to be tested and differences in positivity thresholds. At present, suspect molecules are tested directly, but the difference still lies in the dilution process(29,30).

2.1.1 Prick tests

They demonstrate the presence of allergen-specific IgE antibodies in the skin mast cells responsible for immediate hypersensitivity (31). In the event of dermatitis or infection in the test areas, the test should be postponed until the lesions have healed. The test is not relevant in conjunction with certain treatments, such as: (32)

- Antihistamines are a source of false negatives. We require you to stop taking them for about a week.
- Corticosteroids and immunosuppressants are also a source of false negatives. A more prolonged withdrawal period is required, depending on the nature of the corticosteroid molecule and the route of administration. This situation is sometimes problematic in certain pathologies where the child is obliged to take corticosteroids on a long-term basis. In our study, a child with asthma was forced to delay skin tests on several occasions because of the frequency of oral corticosteroid treatments received for these exacerbations.
- Certain drugs, such as anti-epileptics and anxiolytics, sometimes interfere with the cutaneous reaction, but cannot be stopped. In such cases, skin reactivity must be assessed by the positive control. In our series, no child was taking any of these medications.

Beta blockers reduce the effectiveness of adrenaline in HSI, putting the patient's vital prognosis at risk. They should be discontinued when skin tests are performed, as there is a theoretical risk of diffusion. In fact, the main risk in performing these tests is the occurrence of locoregional or even general diffusion, which is exceptional but always possible. This risk is why these tests should be carried out in a hospital facility capable of handling severe reactions such as anaphylactic shock, with a safety infusion and regular monitoring of vital signs. (17) In our series, an asthma attack was triggered by skin testing in a child with known asthma. It was controlled by nebulized bronchodilators, IV dexamethasone and oral antihistamines. The hemodynamic state was stable, so adrenaline was not justified.

In practical terms, the prick test is performed by placing a drop of the allergen on the forearm or back. A standardized needle is then used to penetrate the drop into the dermis. The test result must be interpreted in relation to a negative control, so as not to overlook dermographism, and a histamine-positive control, to test for cutaneous reactivity. (14,24)

For our patients, dilutions were made manually on the day of testing. For example, the maximum dose recommended by ENDA (48) is 20 of amoxicillin. In practice, dilutions are made to the nearest tenth, and depending on the severity of the immediate reaction, the operator can decide which concentration to start with. For example, if the reaction is severe, lower dilutions will be used as a first step: 20 mg/ml, then 200 mg/ml if the first test is negative.

After around twenty minutes, the test is interpreted by assessing both the papule and the erythema. The test is considered positive if the papule exceeds 3mm (33).

In cases of delayed allergic reaction, it may be possible to take a delayed reading at 48 hours. The test is positive when an eczematous lesion appears at the site of the sting (17,33).

It should be noted that the choice of betalactamine to be tested also depends on the severity of the reaction: in the case of a severe reaction, tests will be carried out for potential alternative molecules from the same family. For common reactions, the molecules consumed will be tested, as well as those with a risk of cross-allergy, and those that could serve as alternatives.

2.1.2. Intradermal reactions

They are only feasible if the molecules to be tested are available in injectable form. This test is useful for exploring immediate and delayed hypersensitivity. RDIs are performed only if the immediate reading of the prick tests was negative. Contraindications and drug interactions are those described for prick tests. The usefulness of a positive and negative control is also justified(34).

This test involves injecting a 0.5 ml volume of allergen into the dermis of the forearm or back. Increasing concentrations are recommended, with the test moving on to the next decimal if the first is negative (33). Interpretation takes about twenty minutes. Positivity is attested by the appearance of a papule over 3 mm with erythema.

A delayed reading after 48 hours can be taken if the incident is more in favor of delayed hypersensitivity. Positivity will be confirmed by the appearance of an eczematous lesion at the site of the sting (34).

TSTs can sometimes be difficult to use in children, due to their varying degrees of pain. In our case, an RID was possible in an 8-year-old girl.

2.1.3. Patch tests

Patch tests explore delayed hypersensitivity. It is the test of choice for maculopapular exanthems (35, 36). In the case of severe reactions, patch tests should be carried out in specialized centers. In addition to the precautions already described for skin tests, this test should not be carried out in cases of phototherapy (37), to avoid false negatives. For example, amoxicillin is tested at a concentration of 30% in petroleum jelly, then applied to the skin under the occlusion of a patch. Readings are taken in two stages, at 48 and 96 hours, or in a single stage with delayed reading. To avoid false positives due to maceration, the reading can be delayed by 3 hours.

The test is considered positive if erythema, vesicles, pruritus and/or edema are observed (17,37).

2.1.4. Diagnostic values

In the investigation of immediate betalactam allergy, prick tests are less sensitive than TSTs. (38).

In the investigation of delayed hypersensitivity, TSTs are also more sensitive than patch tests (39).

To better assess the contribution of skin tests, it was necessary to perform oral reintroduction tests on patients labelled positive, and of course such a practice was not devoid of risk, which posed an ethical problem (39). For this reason, the positive predictive value was not studied, whereas the negative predictive value was well studied. For example, for penicillins, the sensitivity of these tests varies from 61 to 100%, underlining the high negative predictive value, whereas their specificity ranges from 27 to 98%, depending on the series (2,39,40).

In our series, an oral provocation test was performed on a single patient who had developed urticaria while receiving amoxicillin, with a negative prick test. This result was consistent with the literature, which emphasizes the high negative predictive value of OPT and prick tests at certain concentrations (2,39,40).

2.2. In vitro testing

Total IgE has no place in cases of beta-lactam allergy. For amoxicilin, for example, sensitivity ranges from 0 to 53%, but specificity can be as high as 100% (42,43).

Leukocyte activation tests are based on the principle that patients' blood leukocytes (basophils in particular), sensitized by specific IgE antibodies, can be activated by the drug when it is added to the survival medium. Many tests exist, but at present they remain limited to the field of research, since they pose methodological difficulties and have not been validated (44).

2.3. Oral provocation tests

The reference test for confirming the diagnosis of drug allergy is still OPT. However, it is only justified if previous investigations have been negative. This test carries a considerable risk, and should only be carried out in a hospital setting, in a specialized center with the material and human resources to ensure resuscitation. The OPT performed in this study was carried out in the pediatric department, with the presence of the pediatric resuscitation team.

A TPO protocol has been produced by the ENDA group (32). This test can be used to confirm hypersensitivity in cases of suspected allergy to betalactam antibiotics with negative cutaneous investigations. This is exactly the indication for the TPO performed in our series.

This test can also be used to check the tolerance of penicillin-allergic patients to other molecules, in order to propose therapeutic solutions, such as their tolerance to cephalosporins.

They are contraindicated in cases of pregnancy, progressive conditions such as poorly controlled asthma, severe hypersensitivity and positive skin tests. (45,46)

2.4. Diagnostic values of TPO

Although the sensitivity of OPT is indisputable, the need for its use remains controversial. Indeed, some authors cite the high cost-effectiveness of skin testing as justification for not using OPT (47,48). In our series, OPT was negative in the same order as skin tests. Other studies (17,40) report positive diagnoses of penicillin allergy with OPT in 30.7% and 17%. Some authors stipulate that with higher concentrations of active ingredient in skin tests, the risk of false negatives will not exceed 5%. Furthermore, the negative predictive value of OPT for penicillins, for example, is between 94% and 100% (49), justifying the authorization of amoxicillin in a patient with a negative amoxicillin OPT, as is the case in our series (50).

III. OVER-DIAGNOSIS" OF BETALACTAM ALLERGY

Many patients are wrongly diagnosed as allergic (51). In our series, too, of the 38 children suspected of having an allergy, only 13.15% were actually allergic, in line with the literature.

Differential diagnoses are mainly infectious in the paediatric population. Indeed, as already explained in the clinical forms, many bacterial and viral infections closely resemble allergic manifestations. In our study, this possibility was raised in more than half the cases.

Among the differential diagnoses to consider in the paediatric population are food allergies. These include cow's milk protein allergy, egg allergy and nut allergy, which are common in the very young. In our series, this possibility was raised in two children who had eaten a food with a high allergenic potential. However, as the average delay between the event and the allergological consultation was quite long (118 days), the accuracy of the information in relation to the food intake was questionable.

IV. INTEREST IN ELIMINATING OVER-DIAGNOSIS

A multicenter Canadian study showed that allergological investigation led to a significant increase in the use of beta-lactam antibiotics in patients initially labeled allergic (52).

Several other studies have demonstrated the role of in-hospital allergological consultation of suspected antibiotic allergies in minimizing the overall cost of hospitalization (53,54).

It should be noted that many doctors avoid prescribing beta-lactam antibiotics on the basis of a simple doubt on the part of the family, even if an allergological investigation has been carried out attesting to the absence of allergy. This result was also demonstrated in a Western study of the behavior of 206 patients and 163 physicians in the event of a negative allergological work-up to penicillins, where 52% of patients were re-prescribed a penicillin, and only 29% of physicians re-prescribed it. (55)

V. FACTORS PREDICTIVE OF THE ONSET OF A TRUE ALLERGY TO BETALACTAMINES

Studies suggest that certain medical conditions may predispose to β-lactam allergies, such as cystic fibrosis or AIDS. Intermittent and repeated administration and the intravenous route are also predisposing factors (56).

The link between the severity of the reaction presented and the reality of the allergy is not clearly established in the literature. For this reason, investigations should be carried out not only for severe reactions, but also for minor manifestations, following the decision trees described above. (57)

Moreover, in this series, allergological investigations, although few in number, were not limited to severe reactions.

VI. LIMITATIONS OF THE STUDY

This study has certain shortcomings:

- Reduced sample size
- The anamnestic data reported by patients (or their relatives) sometimes lack precision.
- Delays in consultation (over a year) can alter the accuracy of reported facts. What's more, such a delay often makes it impossible to rule out with certainty differential diagnoses, particularly infectious ones, which are fairly common in the paediatric population.
- The distinction between immediate and delayed hypersensitivity was essentially based on the time to onset of symptoms, although this was not precise enough in many cases, probably due to long consultation times.
- The variability of the imputability score reader: although this score is standardized, the subjective element has not been completely eliminated. Indeed, the understanding and interpretation of the facts reported by children or their parents may vary from one investigator to another, while the pharmacological interview in this population was not always carried out by the same person.
- The variability of the imputability score reader could lead to divergent attitudes and final decisions regarding the need or otherwise for allergological investigation. Similarly, the positive diagnosis of an allergy through the history alone could be inaccurate. In this case, allergological investigation was requested by some investigators, but not

by others. This discrepancy is certainly explained by the patients' allergic history, and the severity of the clinical picture, but could also be explained by the subjective interpretation of the facts, and the logistical possibilities of doing or not doing the allergological investigation at the time of the consultation. These discrepancies could ultimately distort the final diagnosis.

- Allergological investigation was indicated in 14 patients, but was only carried out in half of them, which skewed the percentage of confirmed allergy compared with the 38 cases of suspicion recruited.

VII. STUDY HIGHLIGHTS

It would be useful to highlight the strong points of this study:

- This study addresses a common problem in the pediatric population
- This study highlighted the possibility of alternative diagnoses to allergies in the paediatric population, such as viral and bacterial infections, food allergies and skin atopy.
- The results of this study encourage pediatricians to re-prescribe betalactam antibiotics when the imputability score is doubtful in the presence of sufficient argument in collaboration with the pharmacovigilance service, given the low frequency of true allergies. These results also encourage them to dare to re-prescribe beta-lactam antibiotics when the results of allergological investigations are negative.

CONCLUSION

Among the most common side effects of drugs are allergic reactions (1). The drugs most often blamed are antibiotics, particularly the beta-lactam antibiotics. The problem is that many patients are wrongly labelled as allergic (2,3). This amalgam of allergy, cross-allergy and false allergy, with all the prescription limitations it entails, poses a growing problem in the paediatric population, which is vulnerable to infection. The aim of our study was to investigate the characteristics of a paediatric population referred to the regional pharmacovigilance service in Sfax for suspected allergy to betalactam antibiotics, listing the immediate or delayed nature of reactions according to chronology and clinical data.

This is a monocentric, cross-sectional, descriptive study based on a population of children consulting the Sfax regional pharmacovigilance service for suspected adverse drug reactions and who had consumed at least one drug from the beta-lactam family. The age limit was 15 years. Exclusion criteria were essentially incomplete records and use of drugs other than beta-lactam antibiotics. Data were collected from the patient's medical record, including socio-demographic data, general pathological and allergological history, drug and food exposures, data concerning the nature of the adverse event, and the results of imputability score calculations. Allergological investigation data were also recorded.

There were 38 children with a M/F sex ratio of 1.53. The mean age of our population was 5.5 years ±3.8. No family or personal history of drug allergy was noted in our population. Only one case of dermographism was noted. There was no documented history of chronic urticaria or food allergy. Atopy was noted in 5 children (13.15%). Asthma was noted in two children

(5.26%). Concerning the adverse event studied, cutaneous signs were the most frequent manifestation in N=32 children (84.2%), followed by respiratory signs in N=4 children (10.5%). Typical urticaria was diagnosed in 20 children (52.6%). Typical maculopapular exanthema was noted in 7 patients (18.4%). Cutaneous involvement involved the whole body in N=28 cases (73.63%). Only one case of angioedema was associated with urticaria. Mottling with cyanosis was noted in a single patient (2.6%). Respiratory discomfort was reported by 4 patients (10.5%). Wheezing was noted in only one case (2.6%).

Neurological signs were present in 3 patients (7.9%), including a chewing reaction and hypertonia in one patient on cefotaxime, accompanied by cyanosis. These were the only signs of stage 3 anaphylaxis in this patient. Digestive signs were noted in only one patient (2.6%), in the form of abdominal pain mistaken for anaphylaxis, with elevated pancreatic enzymes in a child on ceftazidime.

Immediate hypersensitivity was reported in N=21 patients (55.26% of the study population). According to the Ring and Messmer classification, the majority of cases were stage 1, with typical urticarial lesions. Stage 2 was noted in one patient, with urticaria and wheezing.

Stage 3 anaphylaxis with cyanosis, mottling, chewing and hypertonia of the limbs was observed in one patient without typical urticaria. In the study population, typical maculopapular exanthema was identified in 7 patients, i.e. 18.4% of cases. With regard to exposure at the time of the adverse event, consumption of a chocolate-type histaminolytic agent on the day of the event was reported in only one patient. Seafood consumption was reported in two children. Medication other than betalactam antibiotics was documented in more than half the cases (N=20, 52.6%). Apart from antibiotics, paracetamol was the most co-prescribed drug in N=8 (21.1%), followed by NSAIDs and corticoids in N=4 (10.5%) each. Antibiotic therapy was prescribed concomitantly with betalactam antibiotics in N=9 patients (23.7%). The most commonly used molecule was vancomycin in 4 patients (10.52%). Amoxicillin was the molecule most frequently used by patients in the study population (39.5%). 3rd-generation cephalosporins were used in 34.2% of cases.

In N=25 cases (66%), the children had received the antibiotic orally. ENT was the most frequently reported reason for prescribing betalactam antibiotics in N=11 cases (28.9%). With regard to chronological imputability, the average time elapsed between the last dose of medication and the adverse reaction was 3.7 hours ±4.03, with extremes ranging from 6 minutes to 12 hours; this time was less than or equal to one hour, indicating an immediate reaction in 4 (31%) patients, and greater than one hour, indicating a delayed reaction in 9 (69%). After symptomatic treatment and cessation of antibiotic therapy, clinical manifestations resolved in 34 patients (89.47%). According to the Bégaud score, chronological imputability was doubtful in N=18 patients (47%), and plausible in N=17 others (45%). It was probable in only two patients. Semiological imputability was doubtful in half the cases (N=19). It was probable in only one patient. Differential diagnoses were evoked in cases of doubtful semiological imputability (S1). These included infection N=21 (55%), allergy to other concomitant treatments N=4 (10.5%), food allergy following seafood consumption N=2 (5.26%), and histaminoliberation in an atopic patient who had consumed chocolate (2.6%). Intrinsic imputability was doubtful in N=25 cases (65.78%). It was probable in only one patient. In 63.15% of cases (N=24), the overall imputability of the adverse drug reaction was doubtful. It was probable in 3 patients (8%). Allergological investigations were carried out in only 6 children (15.78%). Patch tests were used to diagnose allergy to amoxicillin + clavulanic acid in one patient, who tested positive for this compound and negative for cefpodoxime and cefuroxime. An immediate-reading TST confirmed a C3G allergy in a girl with a dubious prick test. A prick test was positive for amoxicillin clavulanic acid and C1G, and inconclusive for C3G. However, given the occurrence of an asthma attack, a cephalosporin TST was not performed, and the test was considered positive where all beta-lactam antibiotics were banned.

Questioning was central to the diagnostic approach in this study. In our series, in cases of doubtful imputability, a decision was taken as to whether all betalactam antibiotics could be reintroduced without further allergological investigation in 16 patients, 12 of whom were authorized to take all betalactam antibiotics, with simple monitoring when taking the drug involved in the current episode, and 4 authorized to take them without restriction. This finding underlines the importance of questioning, which enables the restriction on prescribing to be lifted, allowing free therapeutic choice without the need for allergological testing.

To distinguish the mechanism of hypersensitivity, the onset time is a precious element. Classically, IHT involves acute urticaria and pruritus, appearing within an hour of taking the drug, and resolving within 24 hours(12, 17). The typical urticarial nature of the lesions in an allergic context is highly suggestive of immediate hypersensitivity. The severity of anaphylaxis requires an allergological work-up (17), which can be summed up in the notion of an asthmatic attack or loss of consciousness, which may sometimes be the only indicators of an anaphylactic reaction. In our series, stage 3 anaphylaxis was not accompanied by urticarial lesions in one child. That said, it should be remembered that, in the case of a mild reaction, non-pruritic skin lesions exclude urticaria by definition. (17). Moreover, in our series, we counted 5 cases of non-specific cutaneous rush due to the absence of pruritus, and the absence of belonging to a particular semiological entity. In these cases, viral and/or atopic origin seemed the most plausible cause. The picture of delayed hypersensitivity is less obvious, given the clinical diversity of toxidermia and the multitude of other possible pictures, the differential diagnoses being mainly infectious in the paediatric population. Indeed, as already explained in the clinical forms, many bacterial and viral infections closely resemble allergic manifestations. In our study, this possibility was raised in more than half the cases.

Among the differential diagnoses to be considered in the paediatric population is food allergy. In our series, this possibility was raised in two children who had consumed a food with a high allergenic potential. However, as the average delay between the event and the allergological consultation was quite long (118 days), the accuracy of the information concerning food intake was questionable.

With regard to the skin tests carried out for our patients, the dilutions of the prick tests were made manually on the day of the test; the maximum dose recommended by ENDA (48) being 20 of amoxicillin. RIDs are only performed if the immediate reading of the prick test is negative for HSI, and of the patch test for HSR (34). TSTs can sometimes be difficult to use in children, due to their varying degrees of pain. In the case of our patients, an

RID was possible in an 8-year-old girl. The OPT performed in this study was carried out in the pediatric ward, in the presence of the pediatric intensive care team, applying the ENDA group's recommendations for good practice (32). This study served as a reminder of the possibility of alternative diagnoses to allergies in the paediatric population, such as viral and bacterial infections, food allergies and skin atopy. The results of this study encourage pediatricians to re-prescribe betalactam antibiotics when the imputability score is doubtful, in the presence of sufficient argument in collaboration with the pharmacovigilance service, given the low frequency of true allergies.

REFERENCES

1. Demoly P. Drug allergies. Médecine thérapeutique / Pédiatrie. 1 Jan 2007;10(1):34-43.

2. Haouichat H, Guénard L, Bourgeois S, Pauli G, De Blay F. Les tests cutanés dans l'exploration de l'allergie à la pénicilline. Revue Française d'Allergologie et d'Immunologie Clinique. Dec 2002;42(8):779-792.

3. Demoly P, Piette V, Messaad D. Diagnosis of drug allergy: which tests and under what circumstances? Apr 24, 2008

4. Vanderlinden P. Skin Reactions to Antibacterial Agents in General Practice. Journal of Clinical Epidemiology. August 1998;51(8):703-708.

5. MacLaughlin EJ, Saseen JJ, Malone DC. Costs of beta-lactam allergies: selection and costs of antibiotics for patients with a reported beta-lactam allergy. Arch Fam Med. August 2000;9(8):722-726.

6. Sade K, Holtzer I, Levo Y, Kivity S. The economic burden of antibiotic treatment of penicillin-allergic patients in internal medicine wards of a general tertiary care hospital. Clinical Experimental Allergy. Apr 2003;33(4):501-506.

7. Blanca M, Romano A, Torres MJ, Férnandez J, Mayorga C, Rodriguez J, et al. Update on the evaluation of hypersensitivity reactions to betalactams. Allergy. Feb 2009;64(2):183-193.

8. C. Ponvert, C. Weilenmann, J. Wassenberg, P. Walecki, M. L. Bourgeois, J. De Blic, P. Scheinmann, Allergy to betalactam antibiotics in children: a prospective follow-up study in retreated children after negative responses in skin and challenge tests, Allergy, 2007.

9. Naïm Ould, Alexis Rybak, Robert Cohen. Penicillin allergy in pediatrics: what is the reality and when should amoxicillin be discontinued? La revue du praticien. 2018, 68(4);355-8

10. Iwona Poziomkowska-Gçsicka, Michal Kurek. Clinical Manifestations and Causes of Anaphylaxis. Analysis of 382 Cases from the Anaphylaxis Registry in West Pomerania Province in Poland.Int J Environ Res Public Health. 2020 Apr; 17(8): 2787.

11. Blanca M, Romano A, Torres MJ, Férnandez J, Mayorga C, Rodriguez J, et al. Update on the evaluation of hypersensitivity reactions to betalactams. Allergy. Feb 2009;64(2):183-193.

12. Andreas J. B. Immediate type drug hypersensitivity: clinical signs, danger signs and pitfalls. Revue Française d'Allergologie et d'Immunologie Clinique. Apr 2006;46(3):279-282.

13. M. Vigan. Epicutaneous tests. Annales de dermatologie et de vénérologie. 2009. 136, 606-609

14. Bousquet P, Demoly P. Les urticaires au cours d'un traitement anti-infectieux : est-il vraiment souvent en cause ? Revue Française d'Allergologie et d'Immunologie Clinique. Apr 2006;46(3):288-294.

15. Ponvert C. Physiopathology and main diagnostic and therapeutic principles of anaphylactic and anaphylactoid reactions. Revue Française d'Allergologie et d'Immunologie Clinique. Dec 2000;40(8):793-803.

16. Laxenaire M-C, Mertes P-M. Accidents anaphylactiques. EMC - Médecine. Feb 2004;1(1):59-69.

17. AUTEGARDEN Elodie. Screening for penicillin allergies in general practice: validation of a simplified decision tree in a reference allergology center.Thèse de doctorat en médecine.Paris 2013

18. C.Ponvert. Main principles of etiological diagnosis of immediate hypersensitivity reactions to drugs and biological substances. Revue Française d'Allergologie et d'Immunologie Clinique. June 2007;47(4):292-297.

19. Blanca M, Romano A, Torres MJ, Férnandez J, Mayorga C, Rodriguez J, et al. Update on the evaluation of hypersensitivity reactions to betalactams. Allergy. Feb 2009;64(2):183-193

20. Veyrac G, Jolliet P. Urticaire médicamenteuse et imputabilité. Revue Française d'Allergologie et d'Immunologie Clinique. Apr 2006;46(3):283-287.

21. Pirson F. Les maladies allergiques: Rôle du généraliste. Louvain médical. 2004 ;123(2): s12-s20.

22. Chosidow O, Herson S, =Department of Internal Medicine. Hôpital Pitié-Salpêtrière. Paris. FRA. Critères d'imputabilité des accidents d'origine médicamenteuse. La Revue Du Praticien. 1997;47(15):1729-1732.

23. Salkind AR, Cuddy PG, Foxworth JW. The rational clinical examination. Is this patient allergic to penicillin? An evidence-based analysis of the likelihood of penicillin allergy. JAMA. 2001 May 16;285(19):2498-505.

24. LEHERICEY Margot.Allergie aux bêtalactamines: devenir des patients après exploration allergologique.Thèse de doctorat en médecine.Caen Normandie.2020

25. Du Plessis T, Walls G, Jordan A, Holland DJ. Implementation of a pharmacist-led penicillin allergy de-labelling service in a public hospital. J Antimicrob Chemother. 2019 Feb 6;

26. Fiszenson-Albala F, Auzerie V, Mahe E, Farinotti R, Durand-Stocco C, Crickx B, et al. A 6-month prospective survey of cutaneous drug reactions in a hospital setting. British Journal of Dermatology. 2003;149(5):1018-22.

27. Barbaud A, Gonçalo M, Bruynzeel D, Bircher A, European Society of Contact Dermatitis. Guidelines for performing skin tests with drugs in the investigation of cutaneous adverse drug reactions. Contact Derm. 2001 Dec;45(6):321-8.

28. Park MA, Li JTC. Diagnosis and Management of Penicillin Allergy. Mayo Clinic Proceedings. March 2005;80(3):405-410.

29. Foong R-XM, Logan K, Perkin MR, du Toit G. Lack of uniformity in the investigation and management of suspected β-lactam allergy in children. Pediatr Allergy Immunol. 2016;27(5):527-32.

30. Blanca M, Romano A, Torres MJ, Férnandez J, Mayorga C, Rodriguez J, et al. Update on the evaluation of hypersensitivity reactions to betalactams. Allergy. 2009 Feb;64(2): 183-93.

31. Jacques Charpin, Daniel Vervloet. Allergologie. médecine sciences flammarion.

32. Aberer W, Bircher A, Romano A, Blanca M, Campi P, Fernandez J, et al. Drug provocation testing in the diagnosis of drug hypersensitivity reactions: general considerations. Allergy. 2003;58(9):854-863

33. Barbaud A, Goncalo M, Bruynzeel D, Bircher A. Guidelines for performing skin tests withdrugs in the investigation of cutaneous adverse drug reactions. Proposed by the Working party of the ESCD for the study of skin testing in investigating cutaneous adverse drug reactions. Contact Dermatitis. Dec 2001;45(6):321-328.

34. Vanessa Chum. Allergological preparations for intradermal testing at Nancy University Hospital. Determination of the direct cost of manufacturing by the in-house pharmacy. Pharmaceutical Sciences. 2015

35. lB. Milpied, A.-S. Darrigade. Intérêt des patch-tests médicamenteux très à distance d'une toxidermie.Annales de Dermatologie et de Vénéréologie. Volume 144, Issue 12, Supplement, December 2017, Pages S142-S143

36. Romano A, Blanca M, Torres MJ, Bircher A, Aberer W, Brockow K, et al. Diagnosis of nonimmediate reactions to beta-lactam antibiotics. Allergy. Nov 2004;59(11):1153-1160.

37. Brockow K, Romano A, Blanca M, Ring J, Pichler W, Demoly P. General

considerations for skin test procedures in the diagnosis of drug hypersensitivity. Allergy. Jan 2002;57(1):45 -51.

38. Sarti W. Routine use of skin testing for immediate penicillin allergy to 6764 patients in an outpatient clinic. Annals of allergy, asthma & immunology: official publication of the American College of Allergy, Asthma, & Immunology. 1985;155-61

39. Torres M-J, Sanchez-Sabate E, Alvarez J, Mayorga C, Fernandez J, Padial A, et al. Skin test evaluation in nonimmediate allergic reactions to penicillins. Allergy. Feb 2004;59(2):219 -224.

40. Torres J, Romano A, Mayorga C, Carmen M, Guzman AE, Reche M, et al. Diagnostic evaluation of a large group of patients with immediate allergy to penicillins: the role of skin testing. Allergy. sept 2001;56(9):850-856.

41. Demoly P, Arnoux B. Biological investigations of drug allergies. Revue Française d'Allergologie et d'Immunologie Clinique. Sept 2004;44(5):450-455.

42. Imnaculada Donna, Maria J Torres, Maria I Montanes, Tahia D Fernandez. In vitro diagnosis testing for antibiotic allergy. Allergy Asthma Immunol Res. 2017, July.9(4):288-298

43. H Chaabane, S Levevre, C Dzviga. Recommandations pour la prescription et l'interprétation des examens biologiques utilisables dans le cadre du diagnostic ou du suivi des allergies, disponibles en France.Partie 4: allergie aux médicaments. Rev Française d'allergologie. 2021. G Model. REAVL-3046

44. Ponvert C. Physiopathology and main diagnostic and therapeutic principles of anaphylactic and anaphylactoid reactions. Revue Française d'Allergologie et d'Immunologie Clinique. Dec 2000;40(8):793-803.

45. 45 Chosidow O, Herson S, =Department of Internal Medicine. Hôpital Pitié-Salpêtrière. Paris. FRA. Critères d'imputabilité des accidents d'origine médicamenteuse. La Revue Du Praticien. 1997;47(15):1729-1732

46. 46.Romano A, Blanca M, Torres MJ, Bircher A, Aberer W, Brockow K, et al. Diagnosis of

47. nonimmediate reactions to beta-lactam antibiotics. Allergy. 2004 Nov;59(11):1153-60.

48. 47 Alan R. Salkind; MD Paul C. Cuddy. Is this patient Allergic to Penicillin? JAMA. 2001;285(19):2498-2505.

49. 48.Solensky R. Hypersensitivity Reactions to Beta-Lactam Antibiotics. Clinical Reviews in Allergy & Immunology. 2003;24(3):201-220.

50. Bousquet PJ, Pipet A, Bousquet-Rouanet L, Demoly P. Oral challenges are needed in the diagnosis of β-lactam hypersensitivity. Clinical & Experimental Allergy. nov 2007

51. M. Thimmesch, K. El Abd. Revue Française d'AllergologieVolume 61, Issue 2, March 2021, Pages 81-86.

52. Demoly P, Piette V, Messaad D. Diagnosis of drug allergy: which tests and under what circumstances? Apr 24, 2008

53. Leis JA, Palmay L, Ho G, Raybardhan S, Gill S, Kan T, et al. Point-of-Care β-Lactam Allergy Skin Testing by Antimicrobial Stewardship Programs: A Pragmatic Multicenter Prospective Evaluation. Clin Infect Dis. 2017 Oct 1;65(7):1059-65.

54. Trubiano JA, Thursky KA, Stewardson AJ, Urbancic K, Worth LJ, Jackson C, et al. Impact of an Integrated Antibiotic Allergy Testing Program on Antimicrobial Stewardship: A Multicenter Evaluation. Clin Infect Dis. 2017 01;65(1):166-74.

55. Modi AR, Majhail NS, Rybicki L, Athans V, Carlstrom K, Srinivas P, et al. Penicillin allergy skin testing as an antibiotic stewardship intervention reduces alternative antibiotic exposures in hematopoietic stem cell transplant recipients. Transpl Infect Dis. 2019 Dec;21(6):e13175.

56. C.-A. Khau, et al. Intérêt d'une exploration allergologique aux pénicillines, Service d'allergologie et dermatologie. Revue Française d'Allergologie.2013 53(3):364

57. C.-A. Khau, A. Vial-Dupuy, H. Gaouar, J.-E. Autegarden, E. Amsler, A. Nissen, C. Pecquet, C. Frances, A. Soria, Intérêt d'une exploration allergologique aux pénicillines, Service d'allergologie et dermatologie, hôpital Tenon, AP-HP, Paris, France

58. Pascal Demoly, Dominique Hillaire-Buys, Nadia Raison-Peyron, Philippe Godard, FrancoisBernard Michel, Jean Bousquet Identifying and understanding drug allergies. Med Sci (Paris). 2003 March; 19(3): 327-336.

APPENDICES

Appendix 1: Sample form

Betalactam allergies in children

Données sociodemographiques:

Nom...prénom...

Sexe...................................origine: urbaine rurale

Date de naissance ....

age..................................ans

ATCD familiaux d'allergie aux bêtalactamines: oui non

ATCD personnels: atopie asthme urticaire chronique dermographisme

autre.................................

Date de survenue de la réaction ....

Survenue de la réaction en ambulatoire ou en hospitalier

Délai entre la réaction et la consultation................................

Alimentation histamino-libératrice: fraise chocolat thon fromages charcuteries

Concernant l'événement allergique

- Motif de prescription
- Voie d'administration du médicament: per os intraveineuse

Intramusculaire (pour la rocéphine) :

- Facteurs confondants :

  autres médicaments: oui non

si oui: AINS paracétamol autre ATB(molécule :)

antihistaminique ADT corticoïdes neuroleptique

autre autre ....

maladie associée: virose (fièvre)

- Antibiotique administré :

amoxicilline amox+acide clav C1G

C2G C3G orale (molécule :)

C3G voie parentérale (molécule :)

PENI G autre

- Sensibilisation antérieure(prise antérieure du médicament) :
- Sensibilisation antérieure(prise antérieure du médicament) :
- Chronologie : Jour combien du traitement /Délai en heure entre la prise du médicament et la réaction............................. (J/H)
- Qualificatif de la réaction: immédiate retardée
- Caractéristiques de la réaction: cutanées systémiques

  Immédiats non immédiats

  - Symptômes cutanés: prurit isolé urticaire réaction exfoliative , exanthème maculo-papuleux, toxidermie

    Durée des Symptômes cutanés:

  - Symptômes systémique type immédiat:

I : Urticaire généralisée, prurit, malaise, anxiété

II: Angiœdème, oppression thoracique, vertiges, symptômes

digestifs (nausées, vomissements, diarrhées, douleurs abdominales)

Avec ou sans les symptômes du stade précédent

III: Dyspnée, sibilances, stridor, dysphagie, dysarthrie, dysphonie, faiblesse, confusion, sensation de mort imminente

Avec ou sans les symptômes des stades précédents

IV : Hypotension, état de choc, perte de connaissance, perte de selles/urines, cyanose

Avec ou sans les symptômes des stades précédents

- Reprise d'une b-lactamine par la suite sans réaction : (molécule :)

Concernant le score d'imputabilité de la pharmacovigilance

Chronologique: C

Sémiologique: S

Intrinsèque: I

Extrinsèque:E

Interprétation globale du score: Douteux, Plausible, Vraisemblable

Décision de la pharmacovigilance: ....

Diagnostic différentiel ....

Concernant les tests diagnostics réalisés

Prick test ☐ résultats...................................

Patch test ☐ résultats...................................

IDR à lecture immédiate ☐ IDR à lecture tardive ☐

résultats...................................

TPO ☐ résultats...................................

IgE spécifiques ☐ résultats...................................

Appendix 2: Ring and Messmer classification (10)

Classification de Ring et Messmer

Grades	*Symptômes*
I	**Signes cutanéo-muqueux** érythème, urticaire, avec ou sans angioedème
II	**Atteinte multiviscérale modérée** signes cutanéo-muqueux ± hypotension artérielle ± tachycardie ± toux, dyspnée ± signes digestifs
III	**Atteinte mono- ou multiviscérale grave** collapsus cardio-vasculaire, tachycardie ou bradycardie ± troubles du rythme cardiaque ± bronchospasme ± signes digestifs Les signes cutanéo-muqueux peuvent être absents ou n'apparaître qu'au moment de la restauration hémodynamique.
IV	**Arrêt cardiaque**

Appendix 3: French drug imputability method (11)

Tableau 1 : Critères définissant l'imputabilité chronologique d'un médicament

Critères chronologiques	
Délai de survenue de l'effet indésirable par rapport à la prise médicamenteuse	Très suggestif *(choc anaphylactique)*
	Incompatible *(délai insuffisant, effet avant la prise de médicament)*
	Compatible *(tous les autres cas)*
Evolution de l'effet indésirable à l'arrêt du médicament (*dechallenge*)	Suggestive *(régression à l'arrêt)*
	Non concluante *(régression retardée, favorisée par un traitement, recul insuffisant, évolution inconnue, médicament poursuivi, lésions irréversibles ou décès)*
	Non suggestive *(absence de régression d'un événement réversible, régression malgré la poursuite du médicament)*
Nouvelle administration du médicament (*rechallenge*)	Positive *(récidive de l'événement à la réintroduction)*
	Non faite
	Négative *(absence de récidive de l'événement à la réintroduction)*

Tableau 2 : Définition du score d'imputabilité chronologique en fonction des 3 critères

	Délai de survenue	**Très suggestif**			**Compatible**			**Incompatible**
	Rechallenge	**R+**	**R0**	**R-**	**R+**	**R0**	**R-**	
Evolution	**Suggestive**	C3	C3	C1	C3	C2	C1	C0
	Non concluante	C3	C2	C1	C3	C1	C1	C0
	Non suggestive	C1	C1	C1	C1	C1	C0	C0

R+ : rechallenge positif, R0 : rechallenge non fait, R- : rechallenge négatif ; C3 : chronologie vraisemblable, C2 : chronologie plausible, C1 : chronologie douteuse, C0 : chronologie incompatible

Tableau 3 : Critères définissant l'imputabilité sémiologique d'un médicament

Critères sémiologiques	
Explication pharmacodynamique (mécanisme d'action)	Evocateur du rôle du médicament ou facteur favorisant
Facteurs favorisants	Autre situation
Diagnostics différentiels possibles	Non
	Oui
Examens complémentaires de laboratoire prouvant la cause médicamenteuse	Positif
	Non fait
	Négatif

Tableau 4 : Définition du score d'imputabilité sémiologique en fonction des 4 critères

		Explication pharmacodynamique ou facteur favorisant			Autres situations		
	Test spécifique	L+	L0	L-	L+	L0	L-
Diagnostics différentiels	Non	S3	S3	S1	S3	S2	S1
	Oui	S3	S2	S1	S3	S1	S1

L+ : test de laboratoire positif, L0 : test de laboratoire non fait, L- : test de laboratoire négatif ; S3 : sémiologie vraisemblable, S2 : sémiologie plausible, S1 : sémiologie douteuse

Tableau 5 : Association des critères chronologiques C et sémiologiques S en score d'imputabilité I

		Sémiologie		
		S1	S2	S3
Chronologie	C0	I0	I0	I0
	C1	I1	I1	I2
	C2	I1	I2	I3
	C3	I3	I3	I4

I4 : imputabilité très vraisemblable, I3 : imputabilité vraisemblable, I2 : imputabilité plausible, I1 : imputabilité douteuse, I0 : imputabilité incompatible

Tableau 6 : Définition du score d'imputabilité extrinsèque

Critères bibliographiques	
B3 : effet notoire / décrit	Référencé dans les ouvrages de référence : dictionnaire des médicaments, Vidal, Martindale, Meyler's Side Effects of Drugs.
B2 : effet non notoire dans les documents usuels	Publié à une ou deux reprises avec une sémiologie différente ou un médicament voisin
B1 : effet non décrit	Non décrit dans la littérature
B0 : effet non décrit	Non décrit après recherche exhaustive dans la littérature

Tableau 7 : Définition des scores d'imputabilité intrinsèque et extrinsèque selon la méthode Bégaud

Imputabilitéchronologique	Imputabilité sémiologique	Imputabilité intrinsèque (d'après C et S)	Imputabilité bibliographique (extrinsèque)
C0 : Incompatible		I0 : Incompatible	B0 : non décrit (recherche exhaustive)
C1 : Douteuse	S1 : Douteuse	I1 : Douteuse	B1 : non décrit
C2 : Plausible	S2 : Plausible	I2 : Plausible	B2 : non notoire
C3 : Vraisemblable	S3 : Vraisemblable	I3 : Vraisemblable	B3 : notoire
		I4 : Très vraisemblable	

C : Chronologique, S : Sémiologique

Appendix 4: Immediate/non-immediate penicillin allergy testing schemes validated by ENDA

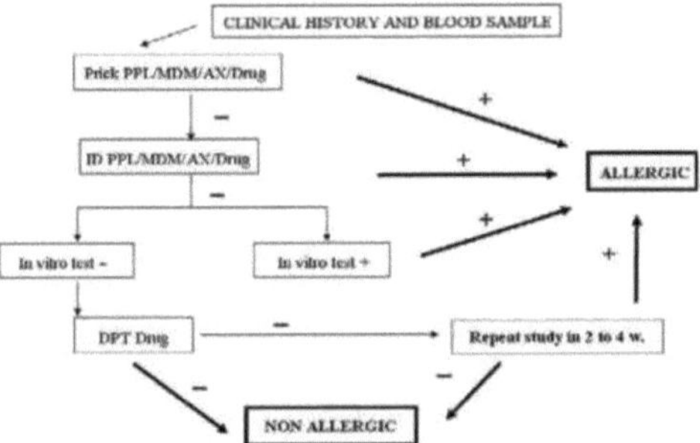

Figure 1. Short algorithm for the diagnosis of immediate allergic reactions to betalactams. This algorithm has the advantage that it can be performed in 1 day and the disadvantage that it fails to distinguish the selectivity of the reaction.

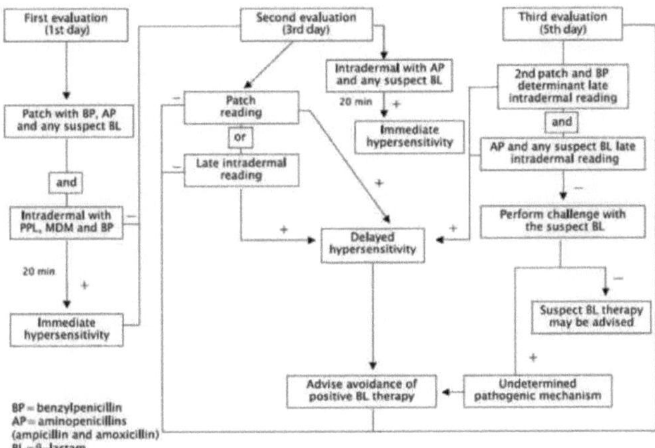

Figure 3. Algorithm for the diagnosis of nonimmediate allergic reactions to betalactams.

Appendix 5: Interview by d'EDNA

ALLERGIE MEDICAMENTEUSE

INVESTIGATEUR :
Nom : .... Centre : .... Date : ....

PATIENT :
Nom : .... Date de naissance : .... Age : ......ans Poids : ......kg
Profession : .... Origine ethnique: .... Sexe : ☐ M ☐F Taille : ......cm

PLAINTES ACTUELLES : ....

Prise art **REACTION MEDICAMENTEUSE :** *1: par rapport au 1er jour* *2: par rapport à dernière prise* 1 2

☐ 1- .... Date de la réaction: .... Chronologie: ....
☐ 2- ....
☐ 3- ....
☐ 4- ....
☐ 5- ....
☐ 6- ....

☐ SYMPTOMES CUTANEO-MUQUEUX:
- ☐ Angioœdème --> localisation : ....
- ☐ Conjonctivite
- ☐ Eczéma de contact ☐ Cause topique ☐ Cause hématogène ☐ ......
- ☐ Exanthème maculeux
- ☐ Exanthème maculopapuleux
- ☐ Erythème pigmenté fixe
- ☐ Prurit isolé
- ☐ Purpura --> Taux des plaquettes: ....
  - ☐ palpable ☐ hémorragique±nécrotique
  - ☐ Atteinte viscérale ....
- ☐ Pustulose exanthématique aigüe généralisée
- ☐ Syndrome de Stevens Johnson / Lyell
- ☐ Urticaire
- ☐ Vascularite urticarienne
- ☐ Autres (préciser morphologie et localisation) :

☐ DIAGNOSTIC DIFFERENTIEL:
....
....

☐ FACTEURS FAVORISANTS:
- ☐ Infections virales : ☐ grippale ☐ Autres
- ☐ Fièvre ....
- ☐ Photosensibilité (lésions photodistribuées) ? ☐Non ☐Oui ☐Ne sait pas
- ☐ Stress
- ☐ Exercice
- ☐ Autres (préciser) : .... ☐

☐ EVOLUTION: *Intensité*

heures / jours

☐ LOCALISATION DES LESIONS ET EVOLUTION (⇑ ⇓, reporter les chiffres ou couleurs différentes si plusieurs réactions)

☐ généralisé

☐ SYMPTOMES GASTROINTESTINAUX:
- ☐ Diarrhée
- ☐ Douleurs gastro-intestinales
- ☐ Nausée, vomissements
- ☐ Autres (préciser) : ....

☐ SYMPTOMES ASSOCIES:
- ☐ Arthralgie/Myalgie --> Localisation/s : ....
- ☐ Douleur/Brûlure --> Localisation/s : ....
- ☐ Fièvre : ......°C
- ☐ Lymphadénopathie --> Localisation/s : ....

☐ SYMPTOMES RESPIRATOIRES:
- ☐ Dyspnée --> DEP ou VEMS : ....
- ☐ Dysphonie
- ☐ Rhinite:
  - ☐ Rhinorrhée
  - ☐ Eternuements
  - ☐ Obstruction nasale
- ☐ Sifflements / Bronchospasme
- ☐ Toux
- ☐ Autres (préciser) : ....

- ☐ Oedème --> Localisation/s: ....
- ☐ Perte de connaissance
- ☐ Autres (préciser) : ....

☐ SYMPTOMES CARDIO-VASCULAIRES:
- ☐ Arythmie
- ☐ Collapsus
- ☐ Hypotension --> Pression artérielle: ....mmHg
- ☐ Tachycardie --> Pouls: ..../min
- ☐ Autres (préciser) : ....

☐ SYMPTOMES PSYCHIQUES:
- ☐ Angoisse / Réactions de panique
- ☐ Hyperventilation
- ☐ Malaise
- ☐ Sueurs
- ☐ Vertige
- ☐ Autre (préciser) : ....

☐ IMPLICATION D'AUTRES ORGANES:
(ex. neuropathie périphérique, atteinte pulmonaire, cytopénie, hépatite...)
- ☐........
- ☐........
- ☐........
- ☐........

❑ **MEDICAMENTS PRIS DEPUIS SANS PROBLEME** :

....

....

....

❑ **MEDICAMENTS SUSPECTES:**

Nom générique du médicament ± additifs / Indication:	Dose quotidienne / Voie Durée du traitement :	Intervalle prise/ réaction	Prise antérieure de ce(s) médicament(s):
1.	......mg/j ....; ....j		❑ Non ❑ Ne sait pas ❑ Oui -> Symptômes: ....
2.	......mg/j ....; ....j		❑ Non ❑ Ne sait pas ❑ Oui -> Symptômes: ....
3.	......mg/j ....; ....j		❑ Non ❑ Ne sait pas ❑ Oui -> Symptômes: ....
4.	......mg/j ....; ....j		❑ Non ❑ Ne sait pas ❑ Oui -> Symptômes: ....
5.	......mg/j ....; ....j		❑ Non ❑ Ne sait pas ❑ Oui -> Symptômes: ....
6.	......mg/j ....; ....j		❑ Non ❑ Ne sait pas ❑ Oui -> Symptômes: ....

❑ Traitement de l'épisode aigü : ❑ Pas de traitement ❑ Consultation urgente ❑ Hospitalisation

❑ Arrêt des médicaments suspectés N° # ....
❑ Antihistaminiques ❑ locaux ❑ oraux ❑ systémiques; --> préciser : ....
❑ Corticostéroïdes ❑ locaux ❑ oraux ❑ systémiques; --> préciser : ....
❑ Bronchodilatateurs ❑ locaux ❑ systémique; --> préciser : ....
❑ Traitement de choc ❑ adrénaline ❑ remplissage vasculaire ❑ autres : ....
❑ Réduction simple de dose de : ....
❑ Changement de médicaments pour : type/nom : .... tolérance : ....
❑ Autre (préciser) : ....

❑ **MEDICAMENTS EN COURS**: ❑ Antihistaminiques: .... ❑ β-Bloquants: ....

❑ Autres médicaments: ....

....

....

....

HISTOIRE PERSONNELLE :

1) Y A T'IL EU DES SYMPTOMES SIMILAIRES OBSERVES SANS PRISE DU MEDICAMENT INCRIMINE ?: ❑Oui ❑ Non ❑ Ne sait pas

....

....

2) ANTECEDENTS :

❑ Asthme
❑ Polypose naso-sinusienne
❑ Mucoviscidose
❑ Diabète
❑ Autre/Préciser :

❑ Autoimmunité (Goujerot, Lupus, etc)
❑ Lymphoprolifération (LAL, LLC, Hodgkin...)
❑ Chirurgie du disque intervertébral
❑ Foie : ....

❑ Urticaria pigmentosa / mastocytose
❑ Urticaire chronique
❑ HIV positif
❑ Rein : ....

....

....

....

....

3) MALADIES ALLERGIQUES: (ex. pollinose, dermatite atopique, allergie alimentaire, allergie aux venins d'hyménoptères, allergie au latex, etc.)

....

....

....

4) REACTIONS MEDICAMENTEUSES LORS DE PRECEDENTES CHIRURGIES (préciser le nombre, avec/sans réaction):

❑ Dentaires: .... ❑Pas de réaction
❑ Anesthésies loco-régionales: .... ❑Pas de réaction
❑ Anesthésies générales: .... ❑Pas de réaction

....

....

....

5) REACTIONS MEDICAMENTEUSES LORS DE VACCINATIONS (oui/non): ❑ Polio ❑ Tétanos

❑ Rubéole ❑ Rougeole ❑ Hépatite B ❑ Diphtérie ❑ Autres: ....

HISTOIRE FAMILIALE :

Allergies / Allergies médicamenteuses : ....

....

TESTS DIAGNOSTIQUES : RESULTATS

1) PENDANT L'EPISODE AIGU:		DATE	NORMAL	ANORMAL	DOUTEUX
Sang:	☐ NFS: ☐ Eosinophiles:	....	☐	☐ Valeur:	☐
	☐ Autres:	....	☐	☐ Valeur:	☐
	☐ ECP	....	☐	☐ Valeur:	☐
	☐ CRP / VS	....	☐	☐ Valeur:	☐
	☐ Cytométrie (.......)	....	☐	☐ Valeur:	☐
	☐ Histamine	....	☐	☐ Valeur:	☐
	☐ Tryptase	....	☐	☐ Valeur:	☐
Foie:	☐ GOT	....	☐	☐ Valeur:	☐
	☐ GPT	....	☐	☐ Valeur:	☐
	☐ γGT	....	☐	☐ Valeur:	☐
	☐ Phosphatase alk.	....	☐	☐ Valeur:	☐
Rein:	☐ Créatinine	....	☐	☐ Valeur:	☐
	☐ Méthylhistaminurie	....	☐	☐ Valeur:	☐
	☐ Autres :	....	☐	☐ Valeur:	☐
Autres:	☐ Médiateurs (IL-4-5-10)	....	☐	☐ Valeur:	☐
	☐ Complexes immuns circ.	....	☐	☐ Valeur:	☐
	☐ Biopsie cutanée	....	☐	☐ Valeur:	
	☐ Complément	....	☐	☐ Valeur:	☐

2) AU DECOURS:		NEGATIF	POSITIF	DOUTEUX
Tests cutanés:	☐ Prick:	☐	☐ Immédiat ☐ Retardé	☐
	....	☐	☐ Immédiat ☐ Retardé	☐
	....	☐	☐ Immédiat ☐ Retardé	☐
	☐ IDR:	☐	☐ Immédiat ☐ Retardé	☐
	....	☐	☐ Immédiat ☐ Retardé	☐
	....	☐	☐ Immédiat ☐ Retardé	☐
	☐ Patch:	☐	☐ Immédiat ☐ Retardé	☐
	....	☐	☐ Immédiat ☐ Retardé	☐
	....	☐	☐ Immédiat ☐ Retardé	☐
Tests sanguins:	☐ IgE totales		☐ Valeur:	
	☐ IgE spécifiques : ☐ CAP ☐ RAST			
	....		☐ Valeur:	
	....		☐ Valeur:	
	....		☐ Valeur:	
	☐ IgG spécifiques/Test de Coombs indir.:		☐ Valeur:	
	☐ Autre:		☐ Valeur:	
Tests cellulaires:	☐ TTL:	☐	☐ SI:	☐
	....	☐	☐ SI:	☐
	☐ Test d'activation des basophiles (préciser : ....)	☐	☐ Valeur:	☐
	☐ CAST:	☐	☐ Valeur:	☐
	☐ Autre:	☐	☐ Valeur:	☐
Tests de provocation:	☐ Anesthésiques locaux :	☐	☐	
	☐ AINS :	☐	☐	
	☐ Aspirine :	☐	☐	
	☐ Paracétamol :	☐	☐	
	☐ β-lactamines :	☐	☐	
	☐ Autres :	☐	☐	

CONCLUSIONS:

☐ Réaction de type I (médiée par les IgE) à : A....................

☐ Réaction de type II (médiée par les anticorps) à : B....................

☐ Réaction de type III (à complexes immuns) à : C....................

☐ Réaction de type IV (cellulaire) à : D....................

☐ Réaction cytotoxique (cellulaire) à : E....................

☐ Réaction pseudoallergique à : F....................

☐ Réaction pharmacologique à : G....................

☐ Réaction psychologique à : H....................

☐ Autre: .... à : I....................

☐ ECHELLE DE PROBABILITE: (marquer la lettre du médicament sur l'échelle)

Très vraisemblable | Vraisemblable | Plausible | Douteux | Exclue / Non cotée

☐ DECLARATION AU CRPV ? ☐ Non ☐ Oui Score : C:......, S:......, I:...... Date: ....

☐ REMARQUES: ....

....

....

Summary

Introduction

Allergy is one of the most common side effects of drugs such as antibiotics, especially betalactamines. The problem is that many patients are wrongly diagnosed as allergic, with all the restrictions on prescriptions that this entails.

Goal

The aim of this study was to investigate the characteristics of a paediatric population with suspected betalactam allergy.

Patients and methods

This is a cross-sectional, descriptive, monocentric study based on a population of children consulting the Sfax regional pharmacovigilance service for suspected allergy to betalactam antibiotics.

Results

The 38 children had a M/F sex ratio of 1.53, with a mean age of 5.5 years ±3.8. Atopy was noted in 5 children (13.15%). Asthma was noted in two children (5.26%). Concerning the adverse event studied, cutaneous signs were the most frequent manifestation in N=32 children (84.2%). Typical urticaria was diagnosed in 20 children (52.6%). Typical maculopapular exanthema was noted in 7 patients (18.4%). Only one case of angioedema was associated with urticaria. Respiratory discomfort was reported by 4 patients (10.5%). Wheezing was noted in only one case (2.6%). Immediate hypersensitivity was reported in N=21 patients (55.26%). Stage 2 anaphylaxis was noted in one patient, with urticaria and wheezing. Stage 3 anaphylaxis with cyanosis, mottling, chewing and hypertonia of the limbs was observed in one patient without typical urticaria. Drug intake other than betalactam antibiotics was documented in more than half the cases (N=20, 52.6%). Apart from antibiotics, paracetamol was the most co-prescribed drug in N=8 (21.1%). Amoxicillin was the most common beta-lactam (39.5%). 3rd-generation cephalosporins were received in 34.2% of cases. In N=25 cases (66%), children had received the antibiotic orally. The average time elapsed between the last dose of medication and the adverse reaction was 3.7 hours ±4.03, with extremes ranging from 6 minutes to 12 hours. This time was less than or equal to one hour, indicating an immediate reaction in 4 patients (31%). According to the Bégaud score, chronological imputability was doubtful in N=18 patients (47%). Semiological imputability was doubtful in half the cases (N=19). It was probable in only one patient. Differential diagnoses were evoked in cases of doubtful semiological imputability (S1), such as infection N= 21 (55%), allergy to other concomitant treatments N=4 (10.5%), food allergy following seafood consumption N=2 (5.26%), and chocolate-induced histaminoliberation (2.6%). Intrinsic imputability was doubtful in N=25 cases (65.78%). It was probable in only one patient. In 63.15% of cases (N=24), overall imputability was doubtful. Allergological investigations were carried out in only 6 children (15.78%), with 1 positive patch test, one positive prick test and one positive IDR. A TPO test was carried out and was negative.

Conclusion

This study highlighted the possibility of alternative diagnoses to allergies in the paediatric population, such as viral and bacterial infections, food allergies and skin atopy. It has encouraged pediatricians to re-prescribe betalactam antibiotics in the presence of sufficient evidence, in collaboration with the pharmacovigilance department, given the low frequency of true allergies.

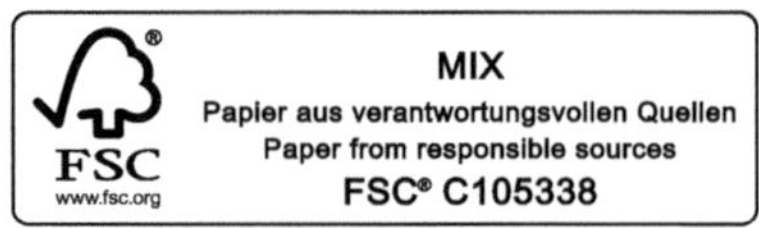

Printed by Books on Demand GmbH, Norderstedt / Germany